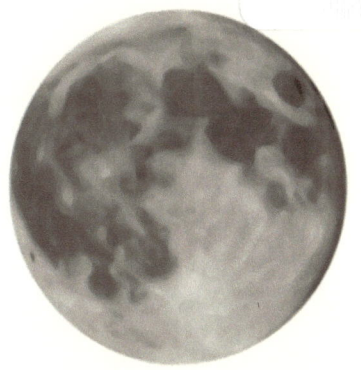

# Sleep

## *The Great Medicine*

### BY ANTHONY CANELO

ISBN: 1492876267

ISBN 13: 9781492876267

Library of Congress Control Number: 2013919749
CreateSpace Independent Publishing Platform
North Charleston, South Carolina

# OTHER BOOKS BY ANTHONY CANELO

The Seven Fundamentals of Longevity

Marriage, Incarceration, Death, Religion & Patience

Self Determination: The Strategy for Mastering Addiction in America

Folk Remedies for the Modern Age

Slowness Gives Wholeness

The Complete Compact Guide to Disaster Survival

The Revival of the Fittest: A Manual to Change the World

Revival of the Fittest: The Prime Material for Human Health and Wisdom

Illustrations by Matthew Mantel

# TABLE OF CONTENTS

Be like the bird who, pausing in her flight awhile on boughs too slight, feels them give way beneath her, and yet sings, knowing she hath wings.

—Victor Hugo

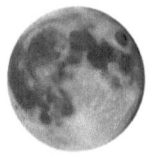

# Introduction

This is not a book about sleep. It is a book about achieving sleep. My primary focus is not on sleep stages, sleep disorders, sleep studies, sleep schedules, or what brain waves are. It is about getting some rest. Sleep-deprived people barely care what scientists may know about sleep. They want restoration. They want a remedy.

I want my readers to discover the all-natural sleep that has them floating at dawn like a drunken god. I want you, the reader, to become madly in love with your dreams. You're going to rise with the morning sun, as long as I have anything to say about it.

Your sleep improvement is a seven-part play. Act one is proper respiration. Acts two and three are nighttime hygiene and hydration. Acts four and five represent attitude and diet. Act six is appropriate exercise. A connection to nature is the seventh act. Your sleep quality is part and parcel to these health fundamentals.

So, let's review the basics. Ask, "How do I desire to spend one third of my life? In comfort? In self-restoration? In sickness and in health? In progress or the past?" It is no surprise that America is fraught with restlessness. The Centers for Disease Control even has a report titled, "Insufficient Sleep Is a Public Epidemic." Three out of every four Americans are getting less than adequate sleep during weekdays.[1] Poor sleep is frequently associated with mood disorders, anxiety, and depression.[2] Even our immune system reacts negatively to sleep disruption. On a night with less

---

1 Reite M., Ruddy J., Nagel K. "Insufficient Sleep Is a Public Epidemic." *Concise Guide to Evaluation and Management of Sleep Disorders* (3rd ed.). American Psychiatric Publishing, Inc., 2002. http://www.cdc.gov/sleep/
2 Better Sleep Council, "Physical Performance & Sleep." www.bettersleep.org,

than five hours of sleep, researchers have proven that our "natural killer cells" decrease in number by nearly 25 percent. That is after only one night![3]

According to Dr. William Collinge, one night of great-quality sleep is more valuable than any health product on the market. I agree. Excellent sleep can increase the natural production of human growth hormone, improve all systems of the body, and extend your life.[4] It can be that easy.

It is puzzling to me how most health professionals offer one or two supplements for sleep improvement. For over a year, I have been wondering why sleep management is not a hot topic. Why are there no famed holistic sleep maximization protocols in the alternative health world? Isn't sleep quintessential natural healing? It is, and so much more than that.

In this book you will learn how to rebuild your nocturnal life from the ground up. I will examine

3 William Collinge. "Sleep's Healing Properties," August 25 1999. www.CNN.com

4 idbg

breathing techniques, food supplements, exercises, beverages, and attitudes that can enhance your rest. You will learn how to mimic REM sleep before you go to sleep. You will learn the incredible roles that calcium and magnesium play in improving your quality of rest. You will find recipes, technology, and plant life that support your resting state. You will even learn how to build your own sleep pyramid.

For each person, health is determined by 'The Seven Fundamentals '. What are '*The* Seven Fundamentals'? In ascending order, they are air, sleep, water, attitude, eating, exercise, and a connection to nature. All together, the seven fundamentals form a quintessential symbol for health and healing: The Phoenix Institute's Holistic Health Pyramid ©.

For me, great sleep is the most enchanting health fundamental. Its barriers are often invisible, yet its success is unmistakable. These remedies are intended for many years of beautiful sleep. I hope and pray they will work for you.

May the remedies herein bring stillness, dividing days.

May sleep become your greatest medicine, in all ways.

*Anthony James Canelo*

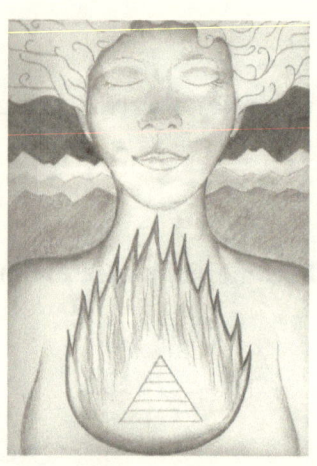

# 'REST'

*"It has been said 'the best things in life are free'.*
*Clearly they were not describing this fire inside me.*
*I have searched the ground to find a roof,*
*pressed wood to earth and stone.*
*In this I found the sacredness of moments spent alone.*
*And when I was alone, laying there, I discovered*
*it was true.*
*The midnight air, all across the sky, kept my flame*
*burning blue.*

*By Anthony Canelo*

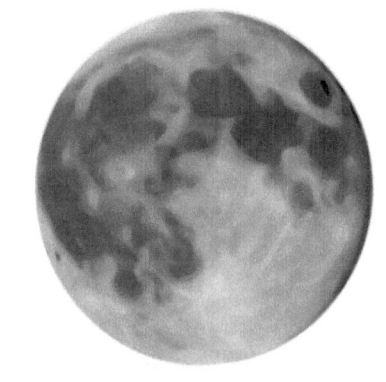

# Breathing

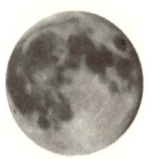

# My Mystic Garden
## Sleep Story

Can you imagine waking up and not feeling tired in the morning? In August 2013 I supported a few of my friends by attending the wonderful Mystic Garden healing arts and music festival in Woodstock, New York. I arrived in a very packed car holding lots of camping equipment. We set up our tents on a difficult incline then danced to incredible live music for several hours into the night. It was an ideal night for dancing, good people, sweet music, and campfires.

Around four in the morning, my dance partner and I were tired. We had not expected it to be so cold and humid that night. Nor did I expect to have our tent lined with odorous mold!

The music was still quite loud outside. After entering our tent, my friend sighed. "I don't know if I'm going to sleep well tonight, Anthony."

Of course, I had other plans. I walked over to my car, reached into the trunk, and pulled out the following items:

2 sleeping masks

2 capes by Martin St. John, made with Polartec fleece

2 sets of earplugs

2 cylindrical pillows

2 handkerchiefs

2 four-foot pieces of rope

1 bag of lavender, chamomile, rose petals, and hops

If anyone was getting sleep that night, it was going to be us.

I returned to my tent with my mouth covered with a wet handkerchief to filter airborne mold, eyes blindfolded, ears plugged, and my body draped with an enormous, soft blue cape. At the inside of my knee, I fastened a small cylindrical pillow with rope. This helped align my back during the night. Perfuming the air with hops and lavender, I hoisted myself into a seated position directly in front of my charmed friend.

She said, "You look like Mothman."

I proposed she become Mothwoman. She casually agreed, draping a long cape over her body just as I had. We were going to sleep on an incline. Therefore I suggested that our heads aim downward to circulate blood to our brains. She agreed. When she was attired properly, I instructed her to breath fifty powerful, deep breaths. After breathing, with aromatic flowers strewn over the pillows and floor, we fell still next to each other like two tired children. We do not know which one of us fell asleep first.

On the one hand, I had slept for only a few hours and rose with the sun, as I am in the habit of doing. I felt sufficiently revitalized. On the other hand, my friend was surprised to have had a full eight hours of sleep. She has told me many times, "It was the best sleep of my life."

She experienced deep, elegant dreams with very little morning fatigue. And, by the way, she forgot to have her usual coffee in the morning. The remedies and perspectives within this book will help you experience the true power of sleep, just like my friend did.

## TAKE A LONG, SLOW, DEEP BREATH

Science says we are carbon-based creatures. Perhaps that is true. However, I like to say we are oxygen-based creatures. Oxygen helps deliver hydration and nutrition. Oxygen stokes the fire of life in every human cell. Without breathing, we die in minutes. A long, slow, deep breath is our most vital and basic connection to life, as everyone knows. When was the last time you took many long, healing, deep breaths? Last night? I'm sure it was. Otherwise you would not be reading this little book today.

The breath is the only automatic health fundamental we have. You can learn a lot from watching healthy children breathe as they sleep. You will notice their expanded and improved muscle action, slow timing, and beautiful consistency. Timing, muscle action, and consistency are elements to keep in mind even while you read this book. As we age, and after many careless breaths, our respiration becomes more restricted and less predictable. If you pay more attention to your wakeful breathing patterns, you can change all of this and improve your nighttime respiration. This chapter will show you how to do just that.

# THE DREAMING MIND AND SENSORY DEPRIVATION

Along with breathing well, it is incredible important to still the mind with a brief concentration exercise.

Of course, the million-dollar question is, "What am I supposed to think about to help me fall asleep?" If you're like me, you've given up on counting sheep a long time ago. Maybe you have also given up on counting backward from one hundred. The following mental exercise is central to sleep management. It is a vitally important method for achieving sleep and will be mentioned many times throughout this book.

Remember, the answer to the million-dollar question is contained within the question itself. What is sleep? Sleep occurs when the brain *shuts off* the body, placing it into a temporary paralytic state via complete sensory deprivation. After achieving paralytic stillness, the brain utilizes a *film reel* of diverse images to heal the body. This "film reel" is also known as the *dream*. Determining the significance of the dream and where it came from is hardly important in your struggle to *achieve* sleep. For our purpose, they are simply random images. When the film reel shows up, we are off into REM (rapid eye movement) sleep, the most healing stage of sleep there is. That is sleep, in a nutshell.

So if you want to sleep more efficiently, you need to concentrate on four principles: paralytic stillness, rapid eye movement, sensory deprivation, and a random sequence of images.

Let's explore these principles with a brief exercise. Lie down and cover your ears and eyes with your fingers or with earplugs and a blindfold. Do not move. Imagine that your brain is starting to send its "shut-down" signals through the body. After several slow, deep breaths, slowly begin to move your eyes at random.

As you breathe, and while your eyes are randomly moving, attempt to access this mental reel of random images. Make an attempt to emotionally surrender to these images that are being produced by your brain, and continue to move your eyes. Concentrate on perfecting this process. Remember to hold your body absolutely still while you access these visual images.

How does this work so well? You are, in effect, mimicking REM sleep. Your eyes are helping to activate the farthest corners of your brain. Your sensory deprivation removes almost all distraction. Your body is shutting down. The film reel begins to get clearer and clearer. If you practice this amazing technique every night, it will get easier and easier. You may soon be able to *listen* for the audio in your film, just as you access its visual elements. I like to call this "rapid ear movement."

This concentration exercise is aligned with the essential qualities of sleep. I call it **REM I**. It will be available to you anytime, with any exercise, and throughout your life.

# POSTURE AND AIR QUALITY

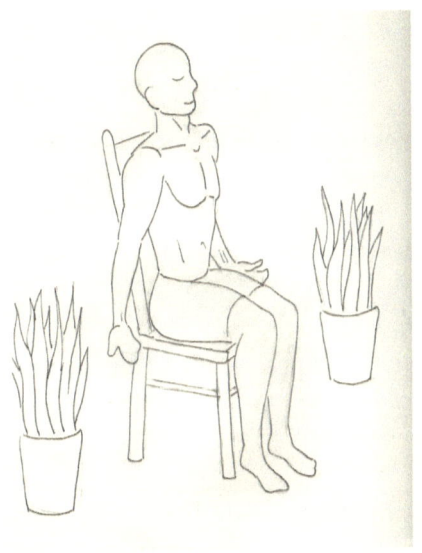

Contrary to popular belief, there is no exclusive benefit from breathing through your nose or mouth. It is much more important to remember that your lungs are roughly the size of a football. If you curl over when you breathe, you constrict your lungs and impede the vital flow of air. So sit up straight, and keep your chin level.

Your lungs are like a muscle. If you use them often, they will get stronger and larger. As they get stronger and larger, you will be able to naturally correct your posture with less effort. The lungs are meant to support the muscles in your back, just as your back muscles are meant to support the expansion of your lungs. Any saxophone player, scuba diver, opera singer, or dedicated breather will agree that a healthy set of lungs can support your body posture. This should motivate you to start a strong breathing practice today and maintain it for the next few days. With practice it will get much easier, just like reading or riding a bicycle.

I have always recommended sleeping with at least six indoor houseplants. Indoor houseplants help to clean your air. They are relaxing, pleasant creatures. Clean air in your room must be a top priority. After all, you will be deep breathing in your room for eight hours per day.

For the sleep-challenged, I strongly recommend you purchase at least twelve snake plants and have them very close to your bed. Snake plants do not require very much maintenance, and they thrive in low light. They are tough little critters. Also, consider purchasing a small twin-blade fan and an ionizer to help move the air in your room and enliven it. You may consider placing a paint strainer bag, filled with activated charcoal, behind the fan. This is a simple trick to help maximize your clean air. If you are considering more intense air purification, I recommend visiting www.iqair.com or www.AustinAir.com.

# THE BREATHING ARTS OF CLEARING AND DISSOLVING

For the purpose of improving sleep quality, there are two distinct categories of breath. The clearing breath is an invigorating, powerful style that can open up the entire respiratory system. It can be done at night, but should always come prior to dissolution breathing.

Dissolution breathing is for deep relaxation. It can slow the heart rate and be done any time. Breathing techniques employing breath dissolution help move us into stillness. All techniques must be accompanied with earplugs, blindfold, and loose-fitting clothes.

**Core Breathing**—Core breathing is a clearing breath. This type of breathing should be done in an upright seated position. Place your blindfold over your eyes. Reach behind your back and place your palms together above your tailbone. Have the tops of your fingers remain touching, as you slowly move apart your palms. Coil the top of your thumbs around each other. Your fingers on each hand should feel very locked together and roughly form an upside-down triangle.

With a perfectly straight back and level chin, inhale deeply, and hold your breath for several seconds. While you hold your breath, tighten your buttocks, lower abdomen, and legs. Be present, and concentrate on centering yourself. Move past unresolved emotional issues. Then, with puckered lips, exhale, making a loud "shhh" sound. Very quickly, inhale again. Repeat this process for about three minutes. You may enjoy an up-tempo song during core breathing. Afterward lie on the ground, and breath in a relaxed manner.

**Vapors**—Breathing vapors are another popular clearing breath. Bring a pot of water to a boil. Fill it with a four bags of chamomile tea, three cloves of garlic, and one large ginger root.

Place a towel over your head and set your face at a comfortable distance from the vapors. Breathe them for at least five minutes. These vapors will help to clean your nasal passages prior to rest. If you do not have a pot at hand, you may soak a handkerchief or cloth in tea tree oil and water, then press this cloth to your face and breathe slowly for several minutes.

**Alternate Nostril Breathing**—This dissolving style of breathing can help you relax and unwind your neurotic thinking. Begin REM I as you are lying down. After a few minutes, close off one nostril with your thumb and inhale completely. Hold your breath for a moment, and then exhale through the opposite nostril. Then inhale through that nostril, and, when ready, exhale through the opposite one. This style of breathing helps to syncopate both sides of the brain. Furthermore, your raised arm will allow more blood to flow to your brain.

**Reverse Limbic Breathing**—This dissolving style of breathing will also help you to unwind and relax. Moreover, it can help you to mimic healthy, nocturnal respiration. To begin, slowly inhale for four seconds and then hold your breath for four seconds. Continue these intermittent inhalations, until you reach the apex of your breath and relax. On the exhalations, shorten your interval period to two seconds. You may breathe in this fashion for several seconds prior to REM I.

# AT NIGHT

For the next few days, make an effort to practice one clearing exercise and one dissolution exercise. Performing them regularly will greatly improve your subsequent dreaming and breathing.

There are many other ways to engage breath work prior to sleep. I encourage you to experiment with yoga or Buteyko breathing as well. Nonetheless, these are my personal choices. I find a combination of breath exercises,

REM I, great posture, and air purification to be the bottom line in helping to improve the quality of your rest.

Feel free to combine these safe suggestions with the other approaches I will offer later in this book.

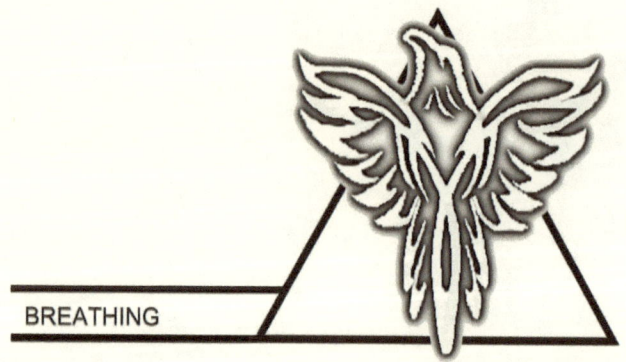

BREATHING

*"Be not afeard. The isle is full of noises,*
*Sounds and sweet airs that give delight and hurt not.*
*Sometimes a thousand twangling instruments*
*Will hum about mine ears, and sometime voices*
*That, if I then had waked after long sleep,*
*Will make me sleep again; and then, in dreaming,*
*The clouds methought would open, and show riches*
*Ready to drop upon me, that when I waked,*
*I cried to dream again."*

— *William Shakespeare*

**The Tempest**

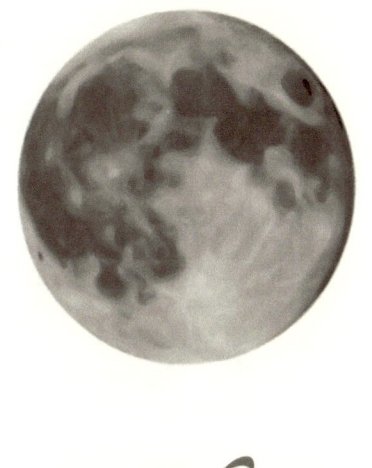

# Sleep

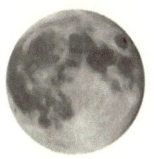

# Unraveling the Causes of Insomnia

How will you unravel that Gordian knot of insomnia? Don't waste time with ineffective medicines. Address the root of the problem: find its cause. For most people sugar, stress, lack of exercise and nutrition, and radiation from television, computers, and cell phones are the top culprits. Electronic screens are addictive and significantly alter brain chemistry. One study found that the more time spent in front of electronic screens, the greater the risk of obesity, chronic diseases, and premature death.[5] Another

---

5  Stamatakis, E. et al. "Screen Based Entertainment Time: All cause mortality, and cardiovascular events: Population based study with ongoing mortality and hospital events followup." *Journal of the American College of Cardiology*, Vol. 57, No. 3, January 2011, pgs. 292–297.

study pointed out that every hour spent in front of television increases your risk of dying prematurely from any by 11 percent![6] Instead of feeding this addiction, one can exercise, eat well, and release stress.

Sugar is another root cause of sleeplessness. Sodas, cookies, and ice cream all contain processed sugar. This highly addictive substance takes a major toll on the body by looting water and oxygen from cells, and frequently causes those disturbing nocturnal blood-sugar spikes. So many people mistake these blood-sugar spikes for over active mental tendencies or an inability to sleep deeply enough! In general, artificial sugars desecrate your body.

Your first priority must be to discover the root cause of your insomnia. Certainly, poor sleep and insomnia are not created by a lack of Ambien, Valium, or other popular medications. Sadly, most medical sleep specialists will have you hooked up to a machine to analyze your brain

---

6 Dunstan D. W. et al. "Television Viewing Time and Mortality: The Australian Diabetes, Obesity, and Lifestyle Study (Ausdiab)." *Circulation*, January 11, 2010.

and body activity before they do deep research on the cause of your insomnia.

Nearly all the time, insomnia is a result of neglecting one or more of the seven health fundamentals. Therefore, the Holistic Health Pyramid is an excellent place to start your search.

A comprehensive detoxification protocol can, in fact, help reverse your restlessness. You may refer to the chlorophyll pollen flower (CPF Fast ©) fast located in the back of this book or arrange to visit your local alternative health professional. Most people sleep much better after a full body cleanse, even if they do not suffer from prolonged insomnia.

## WINDING DOWN

Other than supporting each of your living fundamentals through deep breathing, hydration, positive attitude, wholesome dieting, adequate fitness, and a comfortable environment, a consistent late-night routine is an excellent practice for achieving sleep mastery.

Most often, people undermine the purity of their rest with inappropriate habits. Once again, these habits include staying on the computer or cell phone at night, using stimulants, late-night meals, sugary snacks, drug use, and obsessive-compulsive habits. Avoid these kinds of late-night habits as you develop a practical winding-down routine.

A successful winding-down routine has three basic elements. They are environmental support, social support, and resolving unfinished business.

## ENVIRONMENTAL SUPPORT

Environmental support is about reaching all five senses. Turn down the lights, or light candles. Sprinkle lavender, hops, or chamomile flowers inside your pillows. Eat a light protein snack to help stabilize your blood sugar. Utilize natural sounds or soft classical music. Wear a soft robe or cloak to bed. Have your pillows arranged comfortably.

# SOCIAL SUPPORT

You may reach out for help from family and friends. Organize group massages, or have a moment for communication. You can even allow two or more of your family members to read to you in bed. Focusing on a story will help your mind to relax and wind down. You also can listen to satellite radio programs that feature storytelling. You may strike up a great conversation with a loved one. Feel free to utilize the list of "Getting to know each other" questions from my book *Slowness Gives Wholeness*. Never include television in your social support. Rather, take some time to get to know someone else. There are many sympathetic poor sleepers in the world today. They can help you wind down.

# RESOLVING UNFINISHED BUSINESS

At times we lose sleep simply because we have not gotten something off our chests. Try not to let the undone or unsaid interfere with your winding-down routine. If your unfinished business simply cannot wait, you can write down what you plan to do. You can arrive at an original answer by the morning by creating the intention to dream about it through the night. To do so, take fifteen minutes to contemplate your dilemma in an environment relatively free of sensory stimulation. While contemplating, exercise your imagination. Imagine feeling tones of light-heartedness and ultimate comfort. Remember to breathe and concentrate. Feel free to set yourself up for REM I.

# THE MYSTIC GARDEN SLEEP MAXIMIZATION PROTOCOL

Do you recall the arrangement I prepared for my friend and me? You can do the same for yourself inside your own home. Each ingredient in the Mystic Garden protocol will work harmoniously together or on its own.

**Sleeping Mask**—After fifteen minutes in total darkness, your brain chemistry will begin to pump more melatonin than serotonin. Melatonin is a vital sleep hormone that most people are deficient in. My favorite sleeping masks are the Sleep Master, the Mind Fold, and Dream Essentials.

**Shea Butter**—Cover your legs, abdomen, or torso with a modest amount of shea butter. The fatty acids in shea butter are a wonderful way to promote relaxation and healing throughout the night.

**Cape by Martin St. John**—In my opinion, no greater comfort exists than wearing this beautiful fabric against your body. However, if this particular brand is too costly, visit your local bath supply store, and find a fabric that you find most comfortable wearing. Your robe can be worn during sleep or while winding down.

**Earplugs**—Earplugs increase the effect of melatonin upon the nervous system. They are inexpensive, immeasurably valuable for city sleepers, and can always be worn with a sleeping mask.

**Rope and Cylindrical Pillows**—Tying a pillow to the inside of your leg is a rather ingenious way to correct your posture at night while you toss and turn. If you cannot find a cylindrical pillow, feel free to experiment with other types of pillows. Do not tie your pillow too tightly, because you might inadvertently cut off circulation in one of your legs.

**Handkerchief with essential oils**—During your winding-down time, you may add one drop of rose oil to a bowl of water, dip your handkerchief inside the water, and wear this cloth over your mouth for a few minutes. In combination with your other winding-down tasks, a handkerchief with essential oils is a highly effective tool for promoting calm.

**Buckwheat Pillow with Rose and Hops Flowers**—The Japanese traditionally use buckwheat grouts inside their pillows to promote relaxation. In addition to the calming scent of buckwheat, I recommend you add two handfuls of rose and hops flowers. You may place them inside the pillow, precisely where you will lay your head.

**Set the mood with Stars on Your Ceiling and Music**—For a final touch of magic, attach glow-in-the-dark stars to your ceiling. Then play a few excellent relaxing tunes.

I strongly recommend anything from Nils Frahm, Claude Debussy, or the Monroe Institute. Make sure to listen to 'Felt' by Nils Frahm, 'Open' by The Necks, and "Clair de lune" by Claude Debussy.

**Chamomile Tea**—You have your sleeping mask on your forehead, a soft and lovely cape on your back, earplugs in your ears, stars on your ceiling, a pillow filled with medicinal flowers, and a special leg pillow waiting on your bed. What more does one need? A hot cup of chamomile tea! Chamomile flowers are famous for their calming qualities. Enjoy!

# THE INSOMNIAC'S COLON CLEANSE

Disease, depression, and even deep discomfort often have their roots in a toxic large intestine. I like to call the colon our biological vacuum bag. It is where all toxic material is inevitably expelled or stored. Others have likened the colon to the root systems of a tree. That is a fair analogy. Our colon absorbs an incredible amount of mineral nutrition. For thousands of years, traditional Chinese doctors have claimed, "Death begins in the colon."

Imagine how it must feel to go to the bathroom and drop over ten times the amount of stool that you normally would. That amount, my friends, is a burden to carry.

To improve your sleep, one of the best things you can do before bed is give yourself a spirulina enema. Not only will you absorb a vital amount of organic magnesium and other nutrients, but also you will save your digestive system loads of energy that can be used to heal your body during slumber.

## YOU WILL NEED:

Spirulina powder

Filtered water or freshly distilled water

An enema bucket kit

Coconut oil

**Instructions:** Clean your syringe thoroughly with hydrogen peroxide and alcohol. Next, lubricate your anus with coconut oil. Then lubricate the end of your enema bucket tube with coconut oil. Fill your bucket with water to the desired amount, adding one teaspoon of spirulina powder. Lie down on your back with your knees raised and the soles of your feet on the ground. Release the valve, inserting the water into the rectum, and then remove the syringe. Retain the water for three to fifteen minutes. You may try inverted yoga positions, jumping jacks, or resting alternate nostril breathing. When you are ready, release the water into the toilet. If you have to release multiple times throughout the process, simply clamp down the valve and do so. Releasing might take a few minutes. Afterward, clean your equipment.

# THE HIGH-FREQUENCY VIOLET RAY

The violet ray is one of the most versatile tools ever used for health and healing. It is a unique electrotherapy once advocated by Edgar Cayce, the 'father' of holistic health in America.  Invented by the infamous Nikola Tesla, its safe and practical applications are, in my opinion, worthy of consideration. It can clean and sterilize water; it can energize and sterilize food; it can clean air; and it can be used on almost any part of the body. A violet ray is great for pain, skin conditions, and systemic circulation issues. It operates by delivering clean oxygen and small doses of ozone into the tissues.

Simply stroke the top of your head and spine with a high-frequency violet ray machine for ten minutes before going to sleep. This will provide the energetic, oxygenated balance you will need to fall asleep and stay asleep. One machine is very easy to use and requires a modest investment, after which there is no maintenance cost. The violet ray is particularly useful in helping to relax the body and clarify the mind. At the Phoenix Institute, I often use two professional-sized models on my guests if necessary. A violet ray can be used to press olive or sesame oil blends into the skin. Make sure you clean your glass tubes completely and avoid damaging the machine. Also, you may feel free to use a high-frequency violet ray in conjunction with other therapies. For more information on the high-frequency violet ray, read my first book, *Folk Remedies for the Modern Age*.

# MASTERING THE NOCTURNAL

Quality of sleep is not determined by the hours you get, the drugs you consume, or the mattress that you purchase. Far too many people believe they are getting good sleep if they merely sleep a certain number of hours. Nothing could be more untrue. In reality, sleep quality is determined by the coherence, clarity, and depth of brain-wave activity. Brain-wave activity is determined by the other six fundamentals of health: respiratory capacity, cellular hydration, physical fatigue, attitude, levels of nutrition, and a supportive environment. Your connection to nature is determined by your five senses or the nervous system. What do you see, smell, hear, touch, and even taste during the night?

There will come a time when all people will be able to properly assess the potency of their sleep. For you, that time is now.

# THREE TARGETS FOR OPTIMAL SLEEP

**Dreams**—How often do you remember your dreams? Moreover, how often do you dream? If your dreams are memorable and somewhat vivid, you can give your brain-wave activity a passing score. Contrary to popular belief, there is no age limit to dreaming. If you do not remember your dreams at all, it is almost certain that your health and well-being are declining. Importantly, some people possess a much greater capacity for dreaming than others. Therefore, your capacity to dream is relative to your overall experience.

**Hydration**—Most people do not know what it feels like to wake up without a dry mouth. Likewise, one significant way to determine if you are hydrated is to wake up *without* a parched tongue. If you wake up without a dry mouth, you may receive a good score for sleep potency.

**Fatigue**—Eliminating morning fatigue is the best target for optimal sleep. Young children innately possess this ability. The rest of us have forgotten what it's like. As a young child, do you recall how you used to run around all day, then woke up the following morning refreshed and eager to pursue the day once more? Eliminating morning fatigue requires strict commitment to each health fundamental. If you are one of the few adults who wake up with almost no drowsiness, then give yourself an excellent score for sleeping potency.

**Note**: During sleep, every ninety minutes the human brain cycles through a series of electrical conditions. This action is called a 'sleep cycle'. If you are over forty years old and wake up every ninety minutes, please understand that this is normal with aging. As we age, our ninety-minute sleep cycles tend to lose their potency. It is possible to reverse this tendency with my sleep remedies. However, there is no reason to feel badly about loss of sleep potency. Just like hair loss, it is simply par for the course.

# SURFACES AND ANGLES

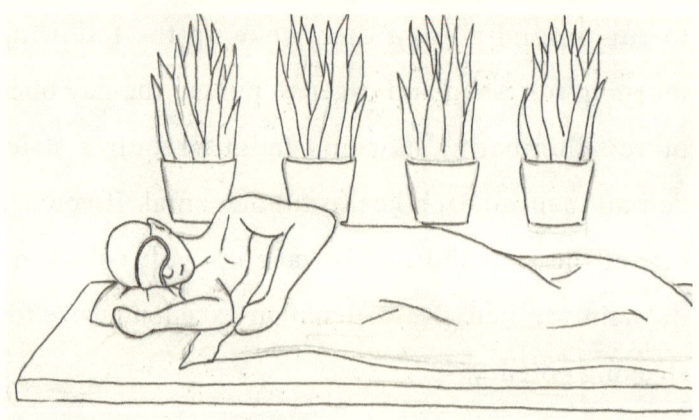

You may find that experimenting with your surfaces and angles of sleep can improve your likelihood of a great night's rest. Start by simply placing something under the midline and far end of your mattress. By inverting your mattress, you flush the brain with blood. You should have your feet propped up at an angle of no more than twenty degrees. Sleep is all about flushing the brain with melatonin. In good sleep, your blood should be rich with melatonin. If you are in the habit of eating before sleep, do not rest on an inverted mattress, as this can cause indigestion.

Explore different surfaces on which to sleep. For thousands of years, human beings evolved sleeping on the ground. This is one of the best options available to you for a more restorative night of sleep. However, there are many people who are not physically capable of trying this. Therefore, you can experiment with sleeping on various surfaces for a while.

You might place a comforter on a hardwood floor. You might also experiment with sleeping on a thick rug. You may need only a small pillow for your face. You can try fitting a pillow between your legs for support if you rest on your side. Each person has a unique and changing body, so experiment on your own by resting on different surfaces.

Every time you roll around on a soft mattress, your body has to compensate for its movement! This is why the people who roll in the night often never stop rolling. Doesn't it make much more sense to sleep on a surface that does not move when you decide to roll?

Often the right angles and surfaces can heal structural problems in very short order! Therefore, experiment with your surfaces and angles for several weeks. Find several angles and surfaces that are particularly comfortable for your body.

# THE POWERS OF INFRARED

If you are fortunate enough to own an infrared bio mat, use it on your legs for half an hour before going to sleep. If you happen to own a full-size infrared mat that you can sleep on, I would say you have made a very wise purchase for your improving your sleep quality.

Infrared heating mats neutralize radiation and provide a wonderful relaxing heat for sleep. Several versions of infrared healing mats have been independently tested and scientifically proven to cancel out all nonionizing radiations. Moreover, infrared light and heat have been shown to improve circulation, support immunity, and improve overall health.[7]

---

7 Lawrence Wilson. *Sauna Therapy* (Prescott, AZ: LD Wilson Consultants, 2004).

# THE PHOENIX INSTITUTE'S RISING TOUCH THERAPY

In February 2012 I invented the Phoenix Institute's Rising Touch Therapy. It is a series of progressive relaxation techniques accompanied by healing technology.

First blindfold yourself. Then perform core breathing for approximately five minutes. As soon as you are finished, lay down on a long infrared heating mat. It should span the length of your body. As you lay there, you may begin the next series of relaxation techniques. Place your ankles atop a 'chi machine', so that your ankles sway from side to side, releasing tension in your spine. Play familiar and relaxing music, and cover yourself with a grounding sheet or bamboo pyramid (refer to chapter 7).

You may accompany this experience with aromatherapy candles. If you have a friend that can help you apply a high-frequency violet ray to your arms, legs, or neck, ask him or her to do so! Your friend will have you sleeping in no time.

I have seen this therapy work near miracles at the Phoenix Institute. Without a doubt, it is the single greatest service in my workshop. It can be replicated anywhere. Even if you do not have all the right equipment, this therapy can still be very effective for deep relaxation and sleep.

# AT NIGHT

You should now have a firm grasp on the importance of winding down. Remember, a winding-down routine is an ever-changing art. Use all that you have available where you may decide to rest. Keep in mind the three targets for excellent sleep.

The technology recommended in this chapter can be found online at Amazon.com. Most of the Mystic Garden sleep-protocol tools can also be found online.

I encourage you to make an investment in your sleep. These technologies will never spoil and will provide you with years of lasting support.

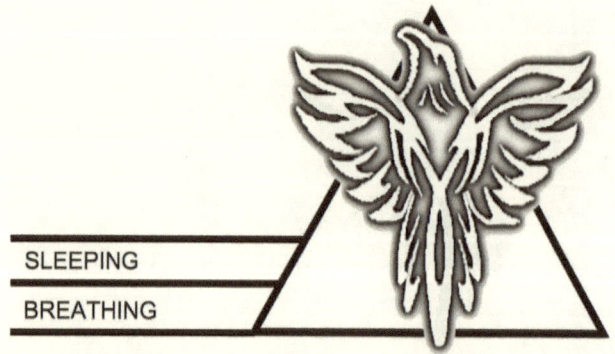

*In rivers*

*The water that you touch is the last of what has passed*

*and the first of that which comes,*

*So with present time.*

—*Leonardo da Vinci*

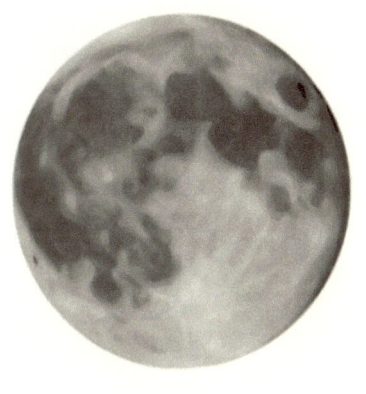

# Water

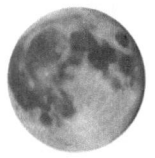

# REM I and the Liquid Cinema

*Transparency, flexibility, crystal clarity, nourishment,* and *flow* are words that convey the magic of water. They can equally convey the magic of sweet dreams. Your brain, body, and dreams are all created with water. Water is the essence of all life.

If you are taking water pills, eating too much salt, or drinking alcohol or caffeinated beverages, you are ruining the balance of your most prized resource. These items are unsafe, principally because they rob or displace the balance of your body's water. Rather than eating too much salt and holding on to waterborne toxins, or draining your water with diuretic fluid, you can preserve your health. Obviously, your sleep would improve very much from this simple advice.

Dehydration is a primary cause for high blood pressure, headaches, muscle pain, and, yes, restlessness. Sodas, coffee, alcohol, and several herbal teas are dehydrating.

A dry mouth in the morning is always a sure sign of dehydration throughout the night. If you are like most people, you wake up with the Gobi desert in your mouth. This, however, is not absolutely necessary. Keep in mind that water breaks down all your nutrition, providing energy for cells, and helps to bond cell membranes. During REM I, when your brain sends its shut-down message to the body, it does so chemically.

In fact, the dream is a liquid cinema. This can explain why the dream brings a buoyant or weightless sensation. During REM I, it helps to notice this.

Our brains are mostly water, as you know. Within this water are a few key ingredients I like to recommend to anyone suffering from insomnia or general restlessness. Calcium, magnesium, phosphorous, potassium, and a pure source of protein are fundamental to the rehydration process.

You should consider purchasing at least three different water filters as well as a stainless steel water bottle for yourself. This will help save you money if you are in the habit of drinking from plastic bottles. It will also protect the environment and radically improve your health. I like recommending one distiller, one high-quality ceramic filter, and one carbon shower filter.

I strongly recommend you find the items I will discuss and keep them in convenient jars alongside your water filter and stainless steel bottle.

# CORAL CALCIUM AND LIQUID MAGNESIUM

When people ask me what my favorite health supplement is, I refer them to coral calcium and liquid magnesium. Calcium itself is the most controversial supplement I know. How well it absorbs, how long it takes to act, its source, and its recommended dosages are hotly contested subjects. They have always been. Calcium represents 85 percent of your mineral need. In fact, several medical doctors have claimed that proper calcium intake can reverse bipolarity, heart disease, sleeplessness, obesity, diabetes, and even cancer.[8] The problem is, proper calcium supplementation is a difficult proposition. Improper calcium metabolism can lead to hypercalcemia!

Nevertheless, calcium is used by all body systems, especially the skeletal and nervous system. Calcium ions travel hundreds of times faster than any other mineral ion and are constantly used to produce neurological activity.[9] It is absolutely imperative to find a trustworthy calcium supplement and to use it frequently.

---

8 Robert R. Barefoot. *Barefoot on Coral Calcium* (Wellness Publishing Co., 2001).

9 Alexander F. Beddoe. *Biologic Ionization* (Warsaw, IN: Whitman, 2002).

I believe what many scientists and doctors have claimed: calcium is the most important health product to consume, and its reputation precedes it. I suggest you start your day with one or two liters of pure water containing liquid magnesium and a coral calcium powder. In nature, calcium is often found with magnesium and many other trace minerals.

I encourage you to find a brand with an excellent reputation and good science to boot. I personally trust New Chapter, Premier Research Laboratories, Life Give, and Barefoot Bob's Coral Calcium. As far as liquid magnesium goes, I prefer the same brands. You may use them at their specified recommended dosages. If you suffer from lack of sleep, you should double your dose. You may double your dose even if you are without sleep issues. Beyond lemon water or coffee, the type of water that contains liquid magnesium has a greater potential to improve the quality of your life. Drink one or two liters in the morning and at least one at night.

Your calcium magnesium-enriched water should taste like very fine mineral water and may have a faded white color to it. Feel free to add spirulina powder to your white water for a far more synergistic effect. I recommend you take all your supplements with this water. This "white water," if used consistently, can provide health improvements well beyond what I have mentioned. Make sure your water is pure, and drink it consistently for at least two weeks. You will start to see results.

# SPIRULINA CALCIUM WATER

**1 liter of pure water**

**Three capsules of 'Barefoot Bob's' coral calcium or**

**add 1/3 teaspoon of alternate calcium powder**

**2 full droppers of 'Health Solute Ions'**

**liquid magnesium**

**2–3 teaspoons of spirulina powder (optional)**

**Instructions: Stir or shake all ingredients together**

# APPLE CIDER VINEGAR AND LECITHIN

Outside of coral calcium and magnesium, granular lecithin and apple cider vinegar are my best recommendations for potassium and phosphorous supplementation. Potassium is an alkalizing mineral used for water control and muscle building. Phosphorous supports the bones, brain health, and the nervous system.

Granular lecithin from soy contains three times as much phosphatidylcholine than eggs, meat, or any other known source. It is not an allergen if obtained from non-genetically modified soy. Lecithin is needed by every cell in our body and comprises 30 percent of the brain's substance. It is universally present in the cells of plant and animal life. Lecithin not only can halt the accumulation of cholesterol, but also it can modulate cholesterol back to normal levels!

Furthermore, it has been proven to reverse senility, clear up skin problems, heal the adrenal glands, clean out arteries, and work as a fabulous preventative for heart attacks.[10] In my practice I have seen lecithin reverse headaches in a matter of minutes. I have also seen it help reverse severe depression, not to mention

10  Carlson Wade. *Lecithin Book,* McGraw Hill, 1998.

obesity and restlessness. I have an incredible affinity for this substance, because it is relatively inexpensive, works profound positive changes in the body, and the results can be seen in a very short period of time. I see it as the great balancer. It helps to balance fat and water levels. It can help balance the sex glands and many other organ/gland systems. It is required for muscle function and maintaining normal weight. For these reasons I give my strongest recommendation for sleepless people to begin supplementing with lecithin.

Lecithin should always be used with vitamins C and E, along with a powerful antioxidant. I recommend super oxide dismutase (SOD) above all else. Here is an excellent recipe:

Olive oil

Uncooked sesame oil

Granular lecithin

Lime

Before working or in the morning, begin by pouring one tablespoon of olive oil and one tablespoon of sesame oil into a cup. Combine them. Then sprinkle two heaping tablespoons of lecithin in this mixture. Juice half of one lime, and drink the lime juice. Follow up the lime juice with this tasty mixture of oil and lecithin. This is also a wonderfully inexpensive way to improve brain function and lose weight.

Apple cider vinegar has also been called a universal health substance. It regularly contains large amounts of potassium, enzymes, calcium, iron, magnesium, beta-carotene, catechins, flavonoids, quercetin, and resveratrol. Its beneficial acids can help digest foods, dissolve fat, and suppress cravings while still being safe for the body's alkaline/acid balance. When processed properly, apple cider vinegar can contain large swaths of beneficial bacteria. This adds to its healing powers.

Apple cider vinegar also promotes the production of hydrochloric acid in the stomach. This can be of extraordinary value for those who suffer from chronic indigestion. If you eat late at night, I recommend you try the following recipe after a meal. It will help you to quickly digest your foods, so that you can enjoy a more complete sleep.

Apple cider vinegar

Raw honey

Bee pollen

In a small cup, pour one to three ounces of apple cider vinegar. Add one-fourth teaspoon of raw honey and one-half teaspoon of bee pollen. Stir this mixture for one minute, until the honey completely dissolves. Drink slowly.

# BLINDFOLDED MELATONIN SUPPLEMENTATION

Melatonin is a very popular sleep remedy and available almost everywhere today. However, a clean brand of liquid melatonin is more preferable than any cheap pill. Liquid melatonin is readily absorbed, gentler on the body, and longer-lasting.

Before REM I, I recommend you practice dissolution breathing for several minutes while blindfolded. After you feel sufficiently relaxed, drink your melatonin supplement without removing your blindfold or earplugs.

This will allow deep sleep to occur very quickly, because you will be mixing both your natural and supplemental melatonin simultaneously.

# SLEEP TONICS

**Passionflower Tonic**—Bring water to a boil. Add two bags of passionflower tea and one-quarter teaspoon activated charcoal. Let cool before drinking. Add catnip extract to this tonic to relax the nervous system.

**Sleepy Time Tonic**—Combine two tablespoons honey, two teaspoons bee pollen, and three teaspoons apple cider vinegar in one cup of freshly boiled water. This is a superb all-natural sleep tonic. Sip slowly.

**Valerian Extract with Kava Kava**—A midnight glass of kava kava tea with valerian extract is an excellent remedy that will help you get to sleep. Valerian extract is a popular natural sleeping remedy, and it can also be added to your cranberry juice. Plus, valerian contains more calcium than any other known herb.

# FOOTBATHS AND BATHS

**Gold Bath no. 1**

Drink a warm cup of passionflower tea while you run a hot bath. When the bath is full, add at least seven bags of chamomile tea. Chamomile is a very popular herb for calming the nervous system. Next, add one-quarter teaspoon of colloidal gold—particularly valuable for enhancing the dream state and providing deep rest—and three drops of essential rose oil. After ten minutes of bathing in this water, add one-quarter cup of conventional 3 percent hydrogen peroxide. You may bathe luxuriously for an additional thirty minutes. This type of bath is a very potent and soothing remedy for restlessness.

**Gold Bath no. 2**

At night steep a cup of passionflower tea while filling a tub for a deeply cleansing, hydrogen peroxide, epsom salt hot bath. You should use one-third cup of good old-fashioned hydrogen peroxide and one-half cup of epsom salts. After you have soaked your body for ten minutes, you may add rose oil and lavender oil to make your bath more soothing and enjoyable. If you are looking for even more gentleness, after fifteen minutes add two drops of jasmine oil and one-half teaspoon of colloidal gold.

Do not fall asleep in the bath! Your bathing should last for no longer than twenty minutes.

**Colloidal Gold Foot Soak**

Frankincense and myrrh are notorious for their soothing anti-inflammatory effects. I have seen frankincense and myrrh foot soaks help soothe gout, arthritis, foot fungus, and warts. Myrrh is a wonderful preservative as well. Once you create a footbath that includes myrrh, the footbath will remain strong for about two days.

Myrrh and colloidal gold are well known for their relaxing effect on the mind.

You may soak your feet for twenty minutes in a tub filled up to your ankles with pure cold or hot water. You may use moderate amounts of both frankincense and myrrh.

Only use less than a teaspoon of colloidal gold in your footbath. A little usually tends to go a very long way.

When combined with earplugs and a short routine of slow breathing, this late-night footbath is most effective.

# THE STRAIGHT CHILLIN' TONIC

My great-tasting Straight Chillin' sleep tonic is so remarkable it deserves a section all its own. It includes a pure source of water, protein, and medicinal herbs

Together, L-glutamine powder and chamomile tea can also help balance blood sugar and cravings for sweets.

To create, add one liter of purified water to a chamomile tea bag, and add two tablespoons of L-glutamine powder. Feel free to double the liquid magnesium for increased relaxation or add your preferred calcium supplement. Enjoy!

# AT NIGHT

The energy in our water is more important than the energy in our food. Water that is subsidized with calcium, magnesium, phosphorous, potassium, and L-glutamine can transform your restlessness into deep calm and balance. So do not get in your body's way, and drain its fluids with coffee, alcohol, and so on.

Starting today set a new goal. Tell yourself, "One day I will wake up in the morning without a dry mouth! That day will be soon!"

Of course, it is absolutely possible.

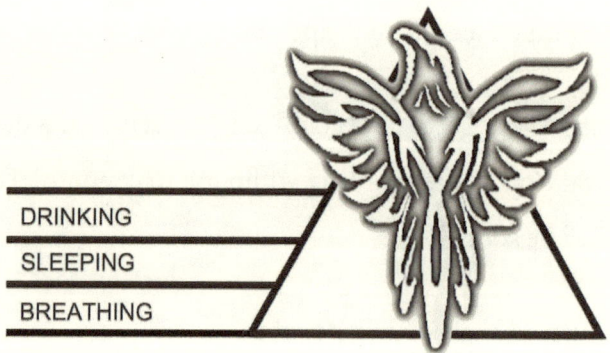

DRINKING

SLEEPING

BREATHING

*Finish every day and be done with it.*

*You have done what you could.*

*Some blunders and absurdities no doubt have crept in;*

*forget them as soon as you can.*

*Tomorrow is a new day; begin it well and serenely and*

*with too high a spirit to be cumbered*

*with your old nonsense.*

*This day is all that is good and fair.*

*It is too dear, with its hopes and invitations, to waste a*

*moment on yesterdays.*

—*Ralph Waldo Emerson*

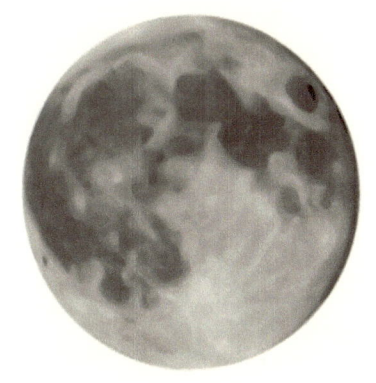

# Attitude

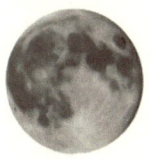

# The Great Indicator

Sleep is the single greatest barometer of attitude. The more you stress, the less you rest. In the past I have recommended cleaning your room, planning your day, writing what you want, tracing works of art, focusing on no thing, the five rhythms practice, reading poetry out loud, reading autobiographies, ways to increase your will to live, and several breathing, concentration, and contemplation exercises. However, in this chapter I will point out the most specific attitude exercises that change your sleep.

Every time we fall into bed and successfully set sail into slumber, we surrender to an unknown experience. This is an experience I cannot claim to comprehend. There are deep mysteries regarding sleep that no scientific person today fully understands. Who is observing the dream? What is the greater purpose of the dream? Where does the observer go during the night? Although the deep magic and mystery of sleep have little to do with *achieving* sleep, it offers clues as to how to unravel the challenges of our fickle attitudes.

Attitude can be your weakest or strongest fundamental. Attitude can be the knife that plunges deep into your heart. Attitude can elevate you to the peak of joy. Yet no matter how painful waking life is, sleep is the great remedy to soothe a weary heart.

# THE ATTITUDE ADVANTAGE OF DREAMING

Here is what we do know about the dream state. Our dreams are often *panoramic*. We have 360-degree vision. Also we experience long moments of *weightlessness*. We might even feel as if we are floating. Third, our dreams are filled with *exaggerated emotions*. Lastly, our dreams represent *deep desires*.

As you do more inner work, remember the advantage of the dream. Wouldn't it behoove you to contemplate your deepest desires? When meditating, must your conscious mind always register linear vision? Must your conscious mind always associate itself with heaviness? In what ways are you conflicted? How do you hold back in daily life?

I suggest you contemplate these advantages as often as you can, particularly before you go to sleep. If you are an experienced meditator, why not introduce the dream's advantages in your practice? You may find they increase mental flexibility and emotional balance. Exercising the inherent faculties of your dreaming mind will help you get to sleep peacefully.

# EMOTIONAL RELEASE

**Vulnerable Confrontation with Slow Feeling**

At the end of the day, your heart may be challenged by emotional fatigue. You can make the decision to clean up your heart and release this fatigue. You need to provide yourself with the right place, the right company, and the right inspiration. You should know that one of the very best ways to get some good rest is to undergo a deep process of emotional release before you go to sleep.

Honor this process. We are all emotional creatures. Sometimes we have to take off a few layers before our naked minds can dream. It is preferable not to have any company if you intend to reach a profound moment of inspiration. Be in a place that is near your bed or close to nature. Perhaps walk outside and enjoy the moon. You may even catch a breeze through an open window. Find your pace to settle down in comfort, wherever it may be.

How we feel before sleep is vital to the healing process. You may have had a good cry, a deep laugh, or an intense moment of stillness before sleeping in your life. How did it feel the morning after? The goal is to re-create that effect, until it becomes second nature. However, your inspiration must be entirely original with every night. After all, who wants to cry and laugh about the same thing night after night? That sounds like a rough breakup to me.

In your place of comfort, you may bring to mind your inspiring theme of the night. It can be sorrow, but make sure that sadness is what you intend to leave behind. It is dangerous to cry tears of self-pity—or to have any pity at all. You want to have your heart and mind filled with emotional wholeness before your rest. Do not cry wandering, blaming, desperate tears. They lead to wandering, blaming, desperate nights. Rather, find tears of joy.

Confronting your vulnerability is the first challenge to emotional release. It is about finding inner suffering that is ripe for transformation into balance, wisdom, and peace. I have several suggestions from my own practice. You might find them helpful.

Celebrate the fact that you now have eight hours to yourself. Celebrate how you feel and how far you have come in your personal healing. Seek out some inspiration. Upworthy.com is a fantastic collection of inspirational videos from all over the world. This website is an incredible resource for extremely joyful and inspirational moments of crying before resting. In addition to upworthy.com, I find speeches by Martin Luther King Jr., Maya Angelou, Steve Jobs, and Randy Pausch to be very inspirational. You may investigate several Tedx speakers as well. Tedx speakers are a beautiful selection of very bright men and women who come from all fields of science, philosophy, art, and more. Start with "Best of Tedx."

What else is beautiful to you? Is it your favorite music? Is it your adored poetry? Perhaps it is a great story from an amazing storyteller. Do you feel that your best days lie ahead of you? Perhaps these items are worthy of your tears. If they are not, find the right inspiration that can guide you to confronting your own vulnerability.

The second challenge of any healthy emotional release is the adrenaline factor. Naturally, when human beings are dealt physical or emotional pain, the tendency is to fight their way out of it or flee (the classic fight-or-flight response). Therefore it is very important to center yourself, slowing both breath and body, and allow your thought to engage your vulnerability—ever so delicately. This is a process I call *slow feeling*. Often we arrive at slow feeling by clearing breath, exercise, or sensual related activities. Slow feeling may be easy for some and extremely difficult for others. If you experience only difficulty, be sure to pick up my book titled *Slowness Gives Wholeness*. Also, slow feeling and slow thinking are always easier once you start to let go and release.

In order to simplify the process of emotional release, let us say that slow feeling (SF) and confronting your vulnerability (CV) bring on emotional release (ER). Here it is in an equation.

$$SF + CV = ER$$

Keep this equation handy. It will help remind you to slow down and search your heart for what you need to find.

# DRAWING YOUR FACE

Improving your imagination will help you to submerge into your dreams with ease. In order to strengthen the faculty of visualization, I suggest you perform the following exercise.

Grab a blank sheet of paper and pen. Then find a mirror, and place it in front of you. Slowly, and with full attention to detail, begin to draw your profile without looking down at the page. If you feel the urge to look down, simply pause and breathe. This exercise is not intended to transform you into a great master of the arts. It is intended to help steady your mind and enhance the visual centers of the brain.

Engage this exercise for at least thirty minutes prior to sleeping. If you find this exercise enjoyable, feel free to make portraits of your family and friends. Drawing faces is an excellent energy outlet for the overactive nocturnal mind.

# ANTICIPATING THE MORNING

Insomnia can be a horrifying experience. To help you decompress, select a certain time of day to perform this next mental exercise.

Lay down with a blindfold and take a few dissolving breaths. For the next twenty minutes, do not move. Begin REM I for only a few minutes. Once you are sufficiently relaxed, imagine the sensation of waking up in the morning. I would like you to experience this feeling with as many senses as possible: visual, tactile, aural, olfactory, and even taste.

The cells in your body do still remember what it feels like to wake up. You probably do as well. Try your best to re-create this feeling in your body.

Once you feel you are locked into this feeling, imagine that you are waking up in tomorrow. Do not take your blindfold off until you register a clear mental impression of waking up rested and healthy. After twenty minutes you may get up and continue with the activities of your day.

# AT NIGHT

The better we feel, the deeper we sleep. In your spare time, ask yourself, "Am I coming to terms with the attitudes reflected in my dreams? What is trying to emerge in my emotional life? Do I explore life as much as I would like to? How do I hold back?"

Emotional release can be extraordinarily satisfying. For some people it comes easily. Others have to work at it daily in order to learn. A good cry, along with exercises to improve your faculty of imagination, can help settle your restless mind.

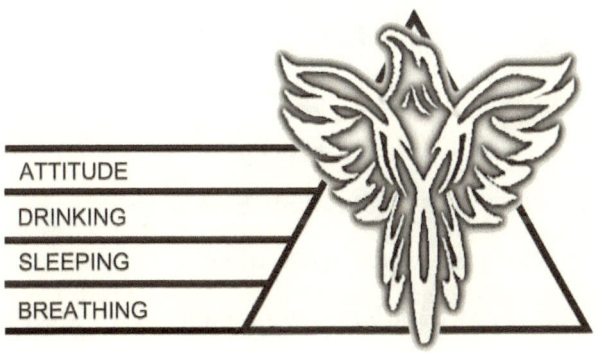

ATTITUDE

DRINKING

SLEEPING

BREATHING

*And when you crush an apple with your teeth,*

*say to it in your heart:*

*Your seeds shall live in my body,*

*And the buds of your tomorrow shall*

*blossom in my heart,*

*And your fragrance shall be my breath,*

*And together we shall rejoice through all the seasons.*

*—Kahlil Gibran*

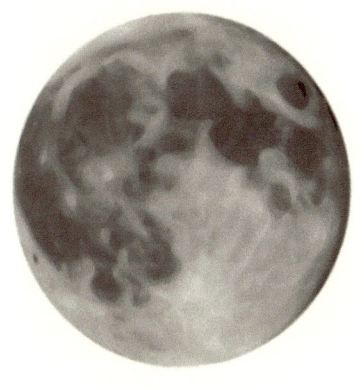

# Eating

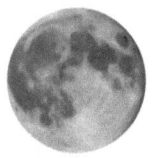

# The SAID Diet ©

Of all seven health fundamentals, eating well is the most endangered. In America, what we eat is often born and raised in a factory, not a garden. The foods we consume are overprocessed and filled with synthetic preservatives, artificial flavoring, and even exogenous hormones that are poisonous. The more you research, the scarier this information about factory foods gets.

As you know, the eating habits of youth are downright silly. Nearly all young people suffer from food addiction, because their parents have very little control over what goes into their mouths. Thus, once a year, young people are enticed to run around in unusual costumes, collecting candy by the pound, while the rates of obesity and childhood diabetes skyrocket past one out of every three children.

The way these young and restless people chose to eat is called the standard American insomniacs diet (SAID©). What should these unfortunate children expect when they grow up? Greater food addiction. Through it all, the sugar industry is the primary culprit; it will lead these badly damaged youth into deeper addiction. Eventually, without properly functioning pancreas, these children will inherit restless nights and seek out alcohol or drugs to quell their blind and chaotic self-destruction.

However, if what people put into their mouths were as important as what clothes they elected to wear, the world would utterly transform in an hour. For you, the reader, it is important to determine your food allergies.

Allergies can be severe. For instance, certain nut allergies can send someone straight to the hospital. However, food allergies can also be very subtle, even unnoticeable. There are two very common food allergies you need to be aware of. They are dairy and gluten. Many people learn they are lactose-intolerant only after a period of abstaining from milk. Reduce your intake of both dairy and gluten, and you might find yourself sleeping better.

Of course, electing to abstain from eating sugar is a no-brainer. This is especially true for those who suffer from severe restlessness. Try living without these foods for a period of eight days, and then see what kind of effect it has on your body when you consume it again.

However, the deeper dilemma at work is food cravings. We all have cravings for foods. Some of these cravings are good, others detrimental. Generally, when out of balance, the body will crave harmful foods. Conversely, when we are properly hydrated, sleeping, stress-free, exercising, and blessed with a connection to nature, our appetite mechanism can right itself to work in our favor.

I have included my popular chlorophyll pollen flower (CPF fast) at the end of this book. The CPF fast supports the realignment of nature's appetite. As a short cleanse, it can help you alleviate your stresses, lose weight, take more-frequent naps, and provide you with powerful knowledge to combat food addiction.

## NO EATING AT NIGHT

Going to bed on a full stomach is like sending your food into a desert to be snatched away by vultures. As long as you are upright, your digestive system can continue to function. In all circumstances, going to sleep on a full stomach severely impedes your body's ability to heal itself.

## FOOD AND SUPPLEMENTS

There is a long list of popular natural sleep-enhancing supplements. These include 5HTP, L-thyronine, magnesium/zinc/B vitamins in combination, GABA, L-glutamine, liquid melatonin, L-tryptophan, L-acetyl cysteine, valerian root, and kava kava. There are food sources for these nutrients, such as pumpkin seeds or pumpkin-seed milk, yellow corn meal, sage, turkey meat, eggs, and lentils.

L-tryptophan is a very important amino acid, because it helps to produce melatonin if metabolized properly. Foods that contain L-tryptophan and its necessary cofactors are almonds, milk, beets, mustard, cucumbers, and turkey.

In my experience working with guests at the Phoenix Institute, I find that non-GMO yellow cornmeal or non-GMO polenta work most effectively when combined with any of the previously mentioned items. If regularly eaten with my apple cider vinegar and bee pollen recipe, this meal will result in a powerful synergy of organic potassium and organic magnesium. Most likely, you will feel it quickly relax the muscles in your body.

# IODINE, SULFUR, MAGNESIUM, PHOSPHOROUS, AND SILICON

These are five food minerals that best aid healthy, deep sleep. I have listed a complete list of foods that are high in these minerals. I encourage you to begin eating them regularly.

**Iodine**—Powdered Nova Scotia dulse, sea lettuce, seafood, carrots, pears, onions, tomatoes, pineapple, potato skins, cod liver oil, garlic, watercress, green leek soup, clam juice, nettle tea. Iodine normalizes metabolism, counteracts poisons, and prevents goiter. Iodine deficiency is indicated by flabby arms, mental depression, or claustrophobia.

**Silicon**—Oats, barley, brown rice, rye, corn, peas, beans, lentils, wheat, spinach, asparagus, lettuce, tomatoes, cabbage, figs, strawberries, rice polishings, oat straw tea, watermelon seeds and rinds, coconut, sage, thyme, hops, prunes, bone marrow, raw egg yolk, pecans, cod liver oil, halibut liver oil. A lack of these foods can cause fragility and hair, skin, or nail problems.

**Phosphorus**—Seafood, milk, raw egg yolk, parsnips, whole wheat, barley, yellow corn, nuts, peas, beans, lentils.

Foods containing phosphorus and foods containing sulfur should be eaten together and are controlled by iodine.

**Magnesium**—Grapefruit, oranges, figs, whole barley, corn, yellow corn meal, wheat bran, coconut, goat's milk, raw egg yolk. Most people are quite deficient in magnesium, which supports bone growth, muscle function, and the nervous system. Magnesium foods are highly recommended for those with excessive emotion, physical tenderness, and excitement problems. Magnesium deficiency has been linked to stress. It has been called "The Relaxer".

**Sulfur**—Garlic, onions, cabbage, cauliflower, asparagus, carrots, horseradish, shrimp, chestnuts, mustard greens, radishes, spinach, leeks, apples, turnips, beet tops, plums, prunes, apricots, peaches, raw egg yolk, melons. Sulfur is needed for brain tissue; it activates the body and intensifies emotion. A lack of these foods can cause depression, poor appetite, or emotional fatigue.

# AT NIGHT

One of the most common causes of sleeplessness is a nocturnal blood-sugar spike. A nocturnal blood-sugar spike is caused by overintake of sugar. Overintake of sugar is caused by a misaligned natural appetite mechanism. In other words, a healthy sleeper has no sweet tooth.

Help your body get the fuel it needs to produce the chemicals that will in turn help bring you into slumber. Remember: to sleep right, eat right.

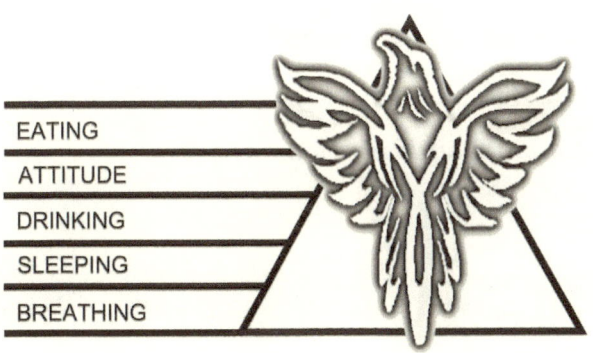

EATING

ATTITUDE

DRINKING

SLEEPING

BREATHING

*Men are born soft and supple; dead they are stiff and hard…. Thus whoever is stiff and inflexible is a disciple of death. Whoever is soft and yielding is a disciple of life.*

—Lao Tzu

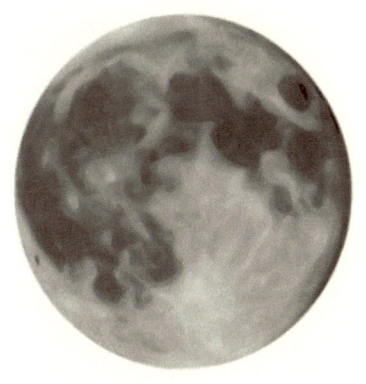

# Exercise

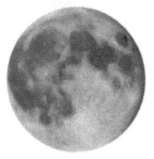

# A Flexible Spine Is a Flexible Life

When it comes to improving your sleep, yoga and massage are therapies of the first order. The tensions each of us holds in our bodies are often overwhelming and interfere with sleep depth as well as overall health. Anyone who has ever experienced one hour of professional massage can testify to this. When was the last time you treated yourself to one?

Of course, moving blood through your feet, legs, back, and neck, clearing out tightness in those areas often has us ready to fall asleep *on* the massage table! No matter the kind of massage, it is an excellent idea to have one regularly, even if you have to do it yourself. In this chapter you will learn a few excellent ways to massage yourself and how to begin an effective home yoga practice designed to promote healthy sleep. Make sure you wear your blindfold whenever possible, and breathe with a purpose.

## INVERTING FOR HEALTH

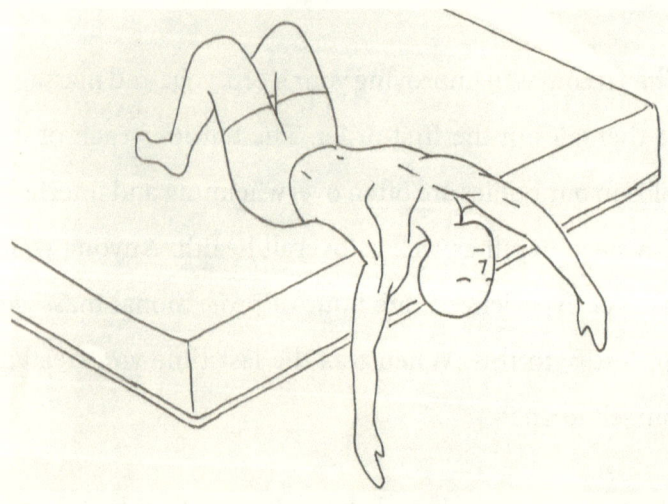

No matter who you are, I recommend you put yourself in an inversion twice daily for two-and-a-half minutes. You may lean off of your bed or stack a few pillows on the wall and slowly walk your legs up the wall while you are in this pose. Try not to feel awkward. This is the time to concentrate. Massage your scalp, and concentrate on breathing deeply. If you have a dry skin brush on hand, begin to massage your torso and arms while you are inverted. You may continue dry brushing for three minutes, then return to a horizontal position for a moment. When you are ready, bring your legs up the wall and begin to massage olive or sesame oil into your thighs, arms, torso, and neck. After a few minutes, you may return to the ground.

This exercise will help you circulate blood throughout your body with astounding effectiveness. It is useful for sleep-deprived folks who do not have the ability to exercise. In performing this exercise, they will receive a similar circulatory benefit.

# BLINDFOLDED STRETCHING FOR SLEEP

There are many safe and effective solutions to help you get to sleep. Stretching your body right before sleep is a superb habit to develop in life. If you have ever been to a yoga class, you may have noticed that your class ended in a resting position. Yogis and yoginis from all over the world agree that Savasana is the most important pose in yoga. Why?

Deep relaxation helps to integrate the work you have done on the mat. It is easy to fall into a deep, trancelike state when you finally enter Savasana. Similarly, sleeping is a way to integrate the experiences of your day. The moment you fall asleep, you begin to reassemble your mind, body, and spirit. So not only does the sacred process of sleep integrate our daily experience, it provides us complete restoration, so that we may live another day.

There is nothing more sacred, beautiful, or gratifying than to wake up and be utterly happy with yourself for no reason. That is what we should strive to achieve in strengthening our most sacred position: the resting position.

# CAT COW AND SINGLE-LEGGED FORWARD BEND

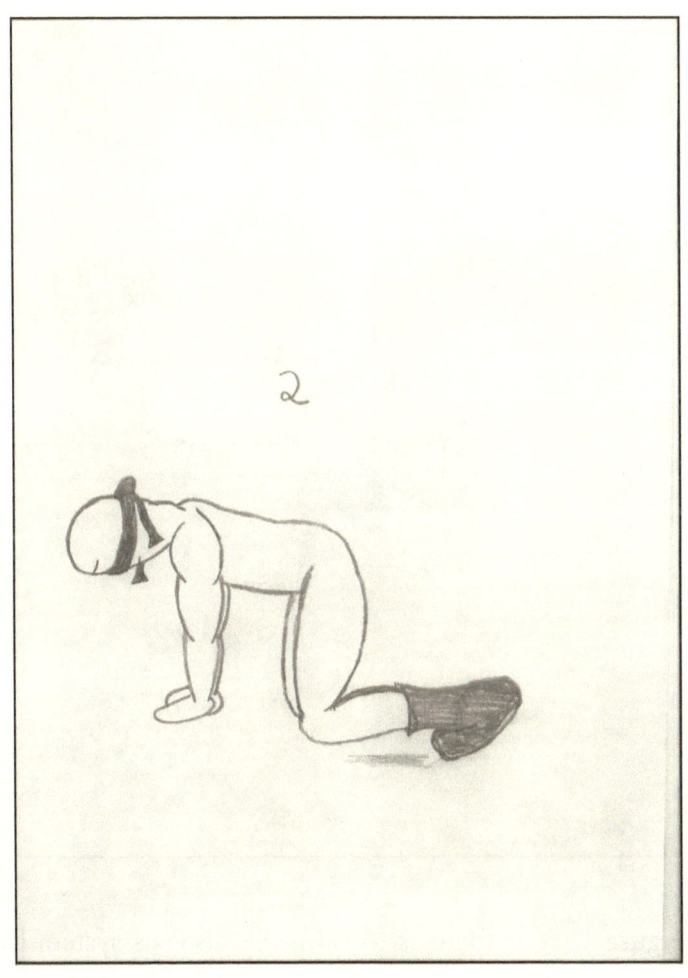

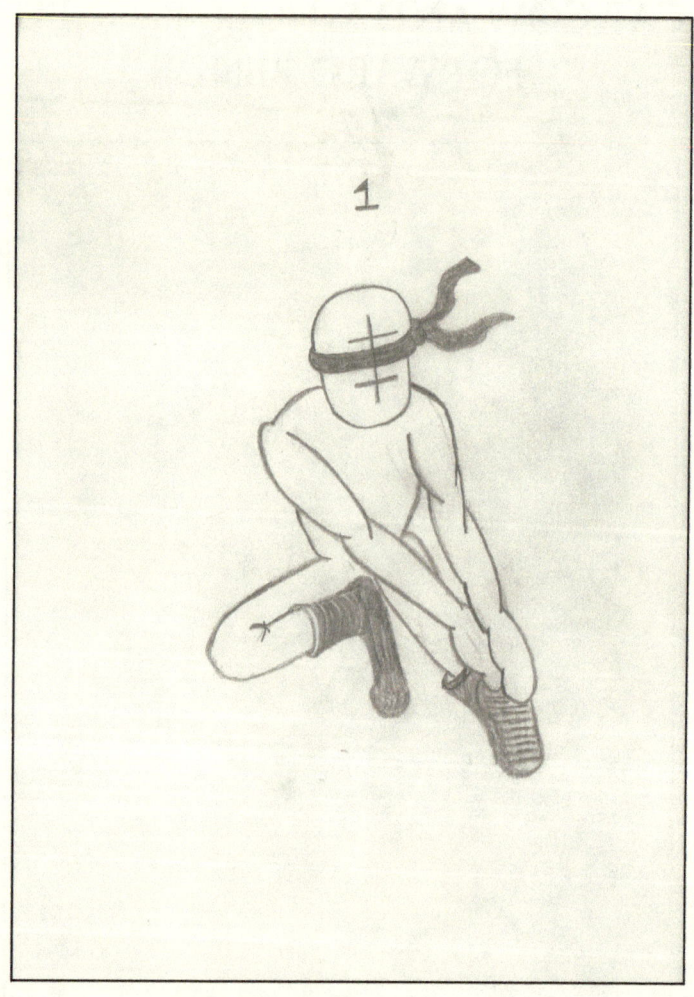

Figure 1. Your focus is to calm the nervous system by gradually decreasing the amount of motion per pose. Remember to blindfold yourself. Then begin by dropping

to your hands and knees. Inhale and lift the head forward, straightening the spine and neck. On your exhale, curl your back upward, like a cat, and tuck your head into your chest. Complete ten repetitions of Cat Cow. Then flip over and sit with your left leg extended in front and your right leg tucked into your inner thigh. Bend over and reach toward your feet. Hold this pose for thirty seconds to one minute, and then switch legs. You may repeat this pose three times per leg.

In general, folding the spine forward tends to calm the nervous system more than any other type of pose. Forward bends are very helpful in relaxing the body before sleep.

# CHILD'S POSE

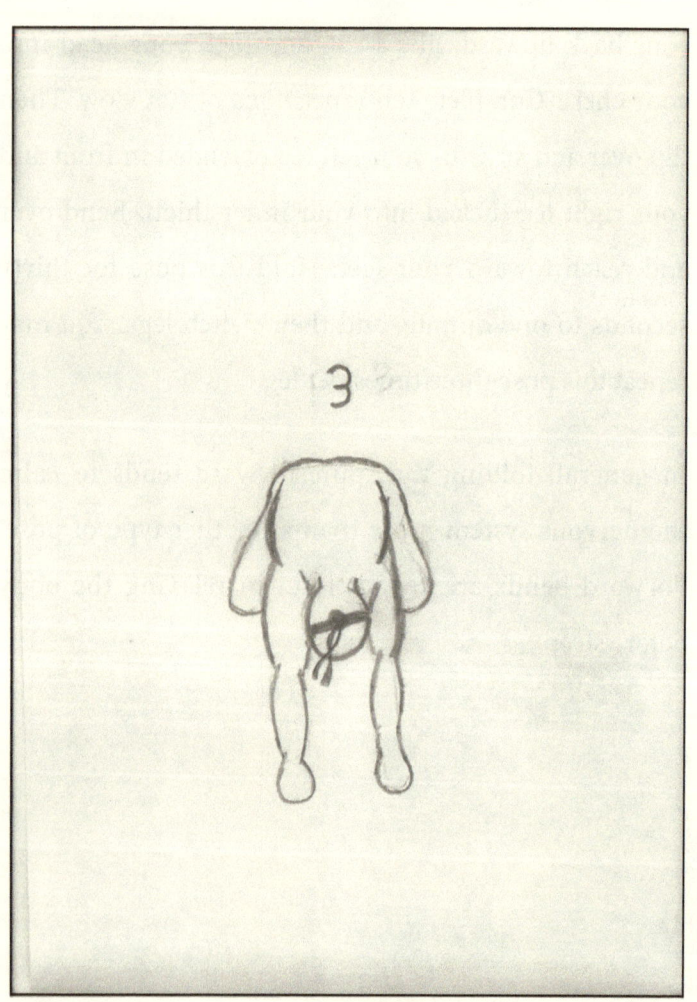

Figure 2. Now you want to take all the stress off your back. Slowly move onto your knees while keeping your shins flat on the floor, with toes touching each other. Sit back on your feet while you reach forward, placing both hands on the floor. Touch your forehead to the floor and remain in this pose for ten breaths. Then turn over onto your back and get into bed.

# SELF-MASSAGING THE MASSETERS AND TEMPORALIS MUSCLES, AND ALTERNATE NOSTRIL BREATHING

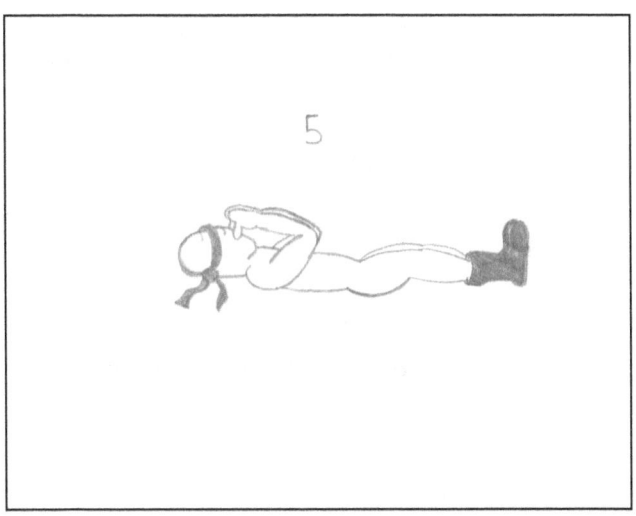

Figure 3. The jaw is the strongest muscle in the body. In fact, our masseter muscles can deliver three hundred pounds of pressure per square inch. Many people have never in their lives released the tensions that build in the jaw. This is why many people who go to sleep stressed tend to grind their teeth at night. Massaging the masseters and temporalis muscles are superb ways to relax the mind as well as an essential part of any healing program. Beginning at the cheekbones, use your thumbs to slowly press along your jaw muscles, while you slowly open and close your mouth in a relaxed manner. After you have massaged your masseters for at least five minutes, you may use your thumbs to work on your temporalis muscles. These are the muscles located between your eyebrows and the top of your ears that bulge when you clench your jaws.

Massage these muscles for five minutes. Remain in a resting position, and begin to breathe in the alternate nostril pattern (as explained in chapter 1).

# AT NIGHT

Please feel free to massage yourself at the end of the day. You can work the larger muscles in your legs with your heels and elbows while still in bed. This can prove an intense and satisfying activity, especially for those restless feet and legs.

It is never a good idea to work out on a partially full stomach. This causes a great deal of added fatigue in the body, because your digestion must work hard to process the last meal. Rather, working out on an empty stomach is preferential.

In general, avoid vigorous exercise before you go to sleep. Light exercise, on the other hand, is acceptable. What is the difference? You are unable to maintain a conversation throughout vigorous exercise.

Vigorous exercise at the end of the day comes with its own health risks. Be careful not to burn the candle at both ends.

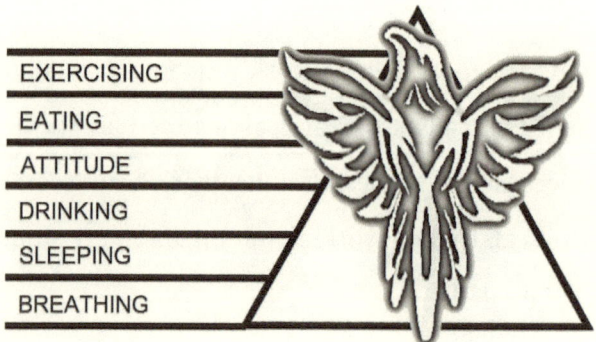

EXERCISING
EATING
ATTITUDE
DRINKING
SLEEPING
BREATHING

*There is a pleasure in the pathless woods,*
*There is a rapture on the lonely shore,*
*There is society, where none intrudes,*
*By the deep sea, and music in its roar:*
*I love not man the less, but Nature more.*

—George Gordon Byron

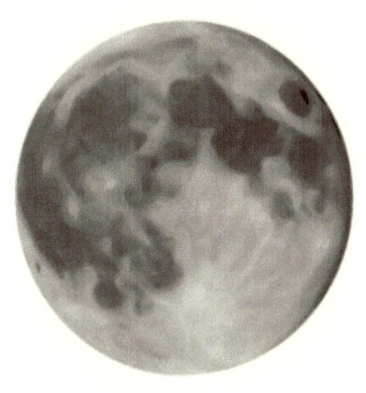

# A
# Connection to
# Nature

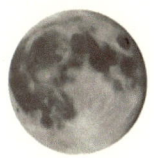

# Chicken-Wire Igloo

Several years ago I was helping my friend record music in his country home. Things were going well, and the house was alive with music. However, after a few hours, it became apparent that there was an enormous amount of static interfering with the electrical instruments. We had to break, while my friend and I attempted to figure out how to solve the problem.

Then, on the suggestion of my friend, I ran into his shed and brought him a large roll of chicken wire. In thirty minutes, we built a massive chicken-wire igloo big enough to house eight musicians rather comfortably. Each wire was buried deep into the ground. It had rained earlier that day, and the ground was moist.

Finally the musicians assembled into the igloo. The moment of truth was fast approaching. Neither my friend nor I were certain that our grounded wires would alleviate the incessant static from the instruments. The musicians turned on their microphones, and we once again were two very happy young men.

The good earth maintains a specific electrical frequency all over its surface. It is known as a grounding force. It is used to help get rid of electrostatic in complex electrical equipment. Also, this force is necessary for all animal life, plant life, weather, and even bacteria. Every time your bare feet touch the ground, you are getting a healthy dose of it.[11] Many researchers, including cardiologist Stephan Sinatra, have testified to its remarkable healing properties. It is also known as vitamin G.

I suggest you follow this fundamental piece of advice. Purchase a grounding sheet, and learn to use it properly. Plug it into a properly grounded wall outlet and it will

---

11  Clint Ober, Stephan Sinatra, and Mark Zucker. *Earthing: The Most Important Medical Discovery Ever?* Basic Health Publications, 2010.

perfectly conduct this healthy, beneficial energy. If you do, you will experience the amazing support of sleeping on the good earth right in your own room. This advice goes part and parcel with the Mystic Garden Protocol, REM I, and the following suggestions within this chapter. Use your grounding sheet often, and use it well.

# THE PYRAMID PLAN©

One look at the Egyptian pyramids, and you know that those fabled Egyptians were up to something deeply cosmic and ingenious. Even with the manpower we have today, some say we probably could not even build the thing. Globally, the Great Pyramid divides the earth into equal parts water and land. It aligns perfectly with true north. It was built in perfect alignment with certain star systems. Its tunneled underground is endless and its architecture harmonically perfected with the natural world. Centuries of mystery surround this structure. It was meant to be more than an entombment. It was a beacon to remind humanity of the great power that lives within. The interesting thing about the great pyramid is its unique power of preservation. If you place rotting fruit inside the king's chamber, it doesn't decay. Nor will a rotting carcass. All living or nonliving biological material appears to be held in suspension. This is the unsung reason why the great pyramids are known the fifth wonder of the ancient world.

*Pyramid* means "fire in the middle." In the king and queen's chamber, visitors have reported everything from personal epiphanies to supernatural phenomena. This has been determined to be true even in smaller, lesser-known pyramids. Many strange things happen inside these famous structures, especially near their centers. Why do these structures have such a "timeless" effect on our perception? Does an invisible mystic fire exist within? It does. Will a pyramid, designed in golden ratios, serve as a bridge to greater thought or greater health? It does. Now, will a portable personal pyramid aid the cognitive process and afford you relaxation, clarity, and rare insights? Yep. They can be easy to build and carry around. Some portable pyramids cost thousands of dollars. I'm going to show you how to make a pyramid, equal in quality, out of bamboo poles and for less than sixty dollars. These pyramids are perfect for individuals hoping to conquer stress, insomnia, and addiction. In my opinion, a bamboo pyramid is a must-have in today's high-stress, fast-paced world.

The golden rectangle is the result of determining the primary mathematical proportions of nature. The ratio of that rectangle's sides is 1.6180339. This ratio is everywhere in nature—from petal to flower, arm to body, and finger to hand. It's the curve ratio of a seashell, the length of your tongue, and it's even displayed in the great arms of the Milky Way galaxy! The design of the cosmos, as well as of nature, is based on this golden ratio. Many believe that aligning any material in golden proportions literally gives life to those materials. To determine the correct height, you must multiply the base (corner to opposite corner) by about .636. You may also decide to just feel it out. As a rule, the closer your pyramid comes to the golden section, the more powerful it will be. Of course, that is not to say it must be exact all the time. For everyday home use, it can be more or less precise, and you will still derive amazing benefits.

The ancient Egyptians believed that the soul itself lived in the center of the human chest, roughly two thirds of the way up the body. Moreover, they believed that the soul animated the body. Of course, any endocrinologist will tell you that a pyramid-shaped gland called the thymus sits right there, in the center of the chest. Interestingly, the thymus gland is closely associated with the aging process and the immune system. Therefore, when you sit in your bamboo pyramid, examine how this part of your body feels. Do you feel your emotional center? Are you in a timeless place? Are you finding clarification? Are you feeling less of an appetite? These are maybe things to ponder on about while inside your personal bamboo pyramid. As you sit in your pyramid, imagine you are sitting within your entire life. Think about your unlimited essence. The healing bamboo pyramid is going to be a movement all over the world very soon. That is, at least, my hope.

Use one material to create your pyramid. I prefer simple bamboo poles. I find bamboo poles work best, because they are cheap and much less denatured than slabs of wood. You can also purchase them in the appropriate five- or six-foot sizes. Remember, you need to build only the frame for the desired balancing effect. Examine my picture. Once you have created the frame of a pyramid, feel free to add any ornamentation. You can draw on it, or you can carve designs on the bamboo—you know, personalize it! The more wood (or homogenous material) you place upon the poles of your pyramid, the more powerful its amplification effect. Be aware that your poles can extend farther than precise measure, just as long as the pyramid form exists in the correct dimensions.

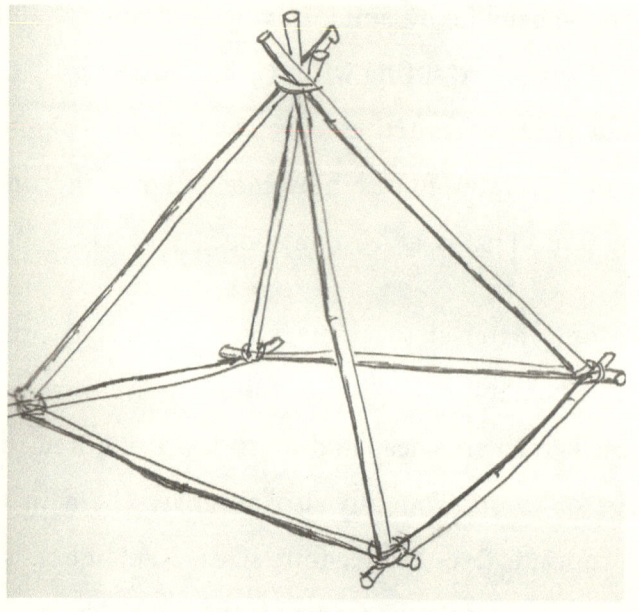

I discourage the use of metallic sheaths or frames; however, I encourage you to place quartz and copper materials in the center. When properly aligned, metal and crystal can properly conduct energy from The Void (a higher mutation of electrical force) rather than cause magnetic interference. To make your personal pyramid nature-friendly, you may stick it into the ground outside. Your outdoor bamboo pyramid will improve the health of your soil, plants, and food crops. You can also place one inside your room and work on your computer while inside—as I am this very moment. This can help keep your mind alert and clear. You can contemplate your next moves from within a pyramid. You may sleep in one. You might eat your meals in one. You could breathe and meditate in one. I urge you to sleep and meditate inside these pyramids. Everyone should have a personal pyramid. It's a no-brainer. They have an uncanny ability to foster emotional and mental clarity.

You can make your own pyramid in less than five minutes, and all these items are found on Amazon.com. They will cost less than sixty dollars in total.

**To set up your own natural lightweight portable pyramid, your will first need to find these three items:**

**24 bamboo poles**

**Twine or rubber bands**

**Optional Items:**

**Moonstone and Rose Quartz (To enhance tranquility)**

**Five quartz crystals (For all purpose amplification)**

**PyraFire mini pyramid (For stronger electromagnetic protection)**

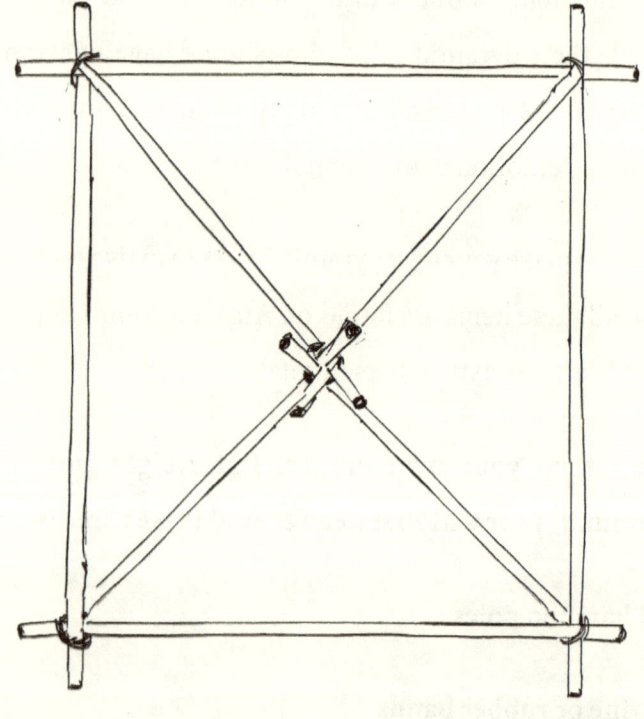

Using twine or rubber bands, group three or four bamboo poles into four separate bundles. These will create a square perimeter.

Again, using twine or rubber bands, group three or four bamboo poles into four separate bundles. Perch each of them in a corner and have them meet in the center. Determine the proper height of your pyramid using a protractor, and measure each corner to exactly 51 degrees. Use a marker to mark the desired height on each one of these bundles. If you desire to use an approximate ratio, or measure it intuitively, feel free. Any approximate pyramid form can produce an effect. I believe the pyramid you make should be appropriately designed for you.

At their point of contact, harness the bamboo poles together with a rubber band or twine.

Your pyramid will likely look like a Native American tepee. That is acceptable, as long as the pyramid form is in existence. You can always build around the pyramid once you have formed the important frame. I would recommend you find out where true north is in your part of the world, and align one of the faces of your pyramid toward that direction. You can sleep in the pyramid facing that direction, also. Some large wooden logs, rocks, or stones to weigh the base of your pyramid down on each corner are a wonderful idea. Cover your pyramid with a black cloth made of natural fibers, and meditate in the darkness. For the ultimate pyramid experience, assemble your bamboo pyramid directly on your grounding sheets, and add one PyraFire mini pyramid (from Premier Laboratories) close to your grounding outlet or directly upon the grounding sheet itself. You can also place one quartz crystal at each corner and at the apex. You can arrange indoor plant life or flowers inside your pyramid. All these suggestions will further amplify the pyramid's energy. The possibilities are unending.

Now you have a very powerful and portable space in which to sleep or learn. So many books have been written on the power of the pyramid forms. I recommend *Pyramid Power* by Patrick Flannagan. I also recommend you listen to "Pyramids" by Ramtha. Conduct your own experiments with unripened fruits! Have a deep rest underneath, and enjoy the "fire in the middle"!

# MY FINAL RECOMMENDATION

Children are often seen hugging pillows. In their innocence, this act represents the ability of a child to cope with loneliness.

If you are struggling for sleep, and living alone, try to find a very large pillow to sleep with at night. Don't be embarrassed. One of my favorite clients calls her large pillow her boyfriend. You do not have to ritualize this touching recommendation. If it feels right to you, just give it a try.

# AT NIGHT

Advancing your REM I practice is what this book is all about. You can enter a small pyramid, cloaked in softness, to enjoy a marvelous glass of kava kava tea as you check out your personal constellations on your ceiling. There are no limits to a life with a deepening attitude, a deepening respect for sleep, and a deepening desire for self-care.

After several years of living by my own suggestions, it has been my sincere pleasure to offer you the best of my knowledge to achieve natural, authentic, inexpensive sleep care. Don't give up on your dreams, and remember that there will always be rest for the weary.

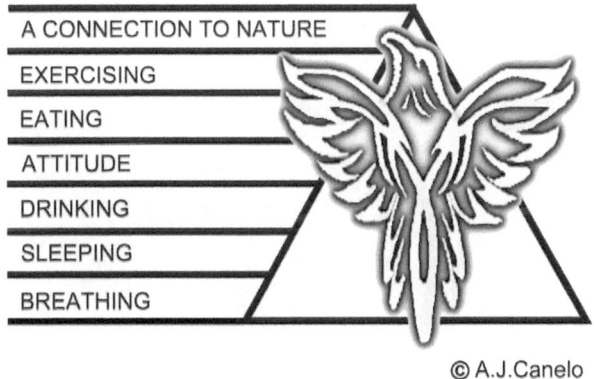

A CONNECTION TO NATURE

EXERCISING

EATING

ATTITUDE

DRINKING

SLEEPING

BREATHING

© A.J.Canelo

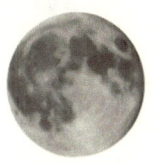

# Purify with the Chlorophyll Pollen Flower Fast ©

I have designed a chlorophyll pollen fast with respect to the body's needs. It is a complete-meal smoothie fast that reduces food cravings and emphasizes sleep improvement. Feel free to engage in REM I, Mystic Garden protocol, and Pyramid Plans at any time during the fast. Enjoy!

**Day 1**

At no later than 2:00 p.m., enjoy a large, healthy salad:

# THIS SALAD HAS THREE MAJOR COMPONENTS

- 70 percent of your large bowl should contain sprouted beans and vegetables.
- A garlic, mustard seed, olive oil, hemp oil, and lemon dressing.
- Sea vegetables, onions, granular lecithin, radishes, kim chi, and sauerkraut may be added for flavor and variety.

**Veggie Sprouts**: Alfalfa, clover, broccoli, snow pea, sunflower, radish, assorted edible flowers

**Bean Sprouts**: Pea, lentil, mung, garbanzo, fenugreek seed

**Sea Veggies**: Whole leaf dulse, nori krinkles, hijiki

**Dressing**: Two parts olive oil, one part refrigerated hemp oil, three juiced lemons, five raw cloves of garlic, and three teaspoons of whole mustard seed. Blend for thirty seconds, until consistency is thick and yellow in color.

**Additional Notes**: Consider purchasing Meyers Green Bags for storing your foods. Make sure you drink at least four glasses of water in the morning. Take a nice walk after you finish eating. This will help to move the fresh, clean blood throughout your body. Forty-five minutes after your meal, drink a green juice or similar beverage high in chlorophyll.

This will be the last meal of the day, so make it large and healthy.

**At 7:00 p.m., prepare Ali's Breakfast Shake:**

2 heaping tablespoons of lecithin granules

2 heaping tablespoons of ground flaxseed

3 heaping tablespoons of protein powder

Blend the above ingredients in 32 oz. of water with two servings of dandelions, kale, lettuce, or broccoli.

*Hemp, rice, and egg protein powder are acceptable substitutes.

**The Pollen and Vinegar Sleepy-Time Tonic:** Before you go to sleep, bring a fresh pot of water to a boil. Add three tablespoons apple cider vinegar, two teaspoons bee pollen, two teaspoons raw honey, and a dash of cinnamon to a large cup of hot water. Drink at least one cup before bed.

## A Cup of Lecithin

Every cell in your body needs lecithin. It helps clean arteries and relieves headaches. Lecithin composes 30 percent of your brain's substance. It will help keep your mind alert, relaxed, and intelligent. It is a universal health substance. Purchase lecithin in granular form from a health-food store. Take three tablespoons in four tablespoons olive or sesame oil. Add lemon juice. Enjoy with a spoon.

## Day 2

Begin this day with twelve deep breaths, a glass of distilled water, and some optional dance, light stretching, or exercise. Play beautiful music then take a hot hydrogen peroxide bath. Stay in the bath no longer than thirty minutes.

**Hydrogen Peroxide Bath**

Add one-half cup of hydrogen peroxide to hot bathwater with one-half cup of charcoal, epsom salt, and apple cider vinegar.

**At 10:00 a.m., prepare a Bee Pollen Breakfast Blend:**

Bring at least thirty-two ounces of purified water to a boil.

Add three tablespoons bee pollen, two tablespoons raw honey, two juiced lemons, and a small pinch of saffron.

Begin Day 2 with this complete protein beverage. The Bee Pollen Breakfast Blend is specifically designed to eliminate food cravings.

**Important:** After you finish your breakfast, enjoy three tablespoons of coconut oil and one tablespoon lecithin over a period of fifteen minutes. Then go for a nice walk.

**Lecithin**

At some time during the day take another three tablespoons of granular lecithin in four tablespoons olive or sesame oil. Add lemon juice. Enjoy with a spoon. This delightful glass of 'brain nutrition' can also help ward of food cravings.

## Jumping Jacks

At some time during the day, do some jumping jacks. Ideally, you should do them until you feel you have broken a sweat. However, go at your own pace. Then sit on the ground and perform limbic breathing. Please remove your shoes, so your feet can touch the earth.

## Grounding

Grounding is important, because physical contact with the earth's telluric field has scientifically proven benefits for human health. These include a normalization of levels of cortisol (the "stress hormone"), c-reactive proteins (inflammation), melatonin (the relaxation hormone), and protection against excessive radiation exposure. The practice is commonly called *Earthing*. Find a tree to lean on if sitting up is difficult. I suggest massaging sesame oil or castor oil on your feet; this will increase your skin's conductivity. Then perform limbic breathing for thirty minutes. If it is too cold outside, you may soak your feet in a charcoal peroxide footbath.

**Activated Charcoal Peroxide Footbath**

Use any plastic tub to submerge your feet. Rubber rain boots are more convenient for this purpose. Fill the water up to your ankles, and add four ounces of peroxide and four ounces of activated charcoal (that is, two ounces of each to each boot). Use distilled water if possible. Charcoal has electrostatic properties that simulate the benefits of Earthing. You may also perform the optional additional instructions below.

**Additional Instructions**

1) In addition to the basic limbic breathing pattern, you can blindfold yourself in order to receive the rejuvenating powers of melatonin. I also suggest listening to your natural environment for further relaxation.

2)    You can engage in mental exercises. Try staring at one point in the distance for the entire length of your limbic breathing exercise. Do not move your eyes from this spot, and begin the process of concentration. This is a great time to engage in all mental exercises.

**At noon, prepare a Blue Nut Milk Smoothie** (If you do not feel like drinking a smoothie, then skip this step.)

**Instructions:** Blend five almonds and five blueberries in at least 32 oz. of water. Continue as if preparing an Ali's Breakfast Smoothie.

**Flower and Vinegar:** Between 12:30 and 5:00 p.m., you may experience food cravings. If you do, fill a small cup with three ounces of apple cider vinegar and one-half teaspoon of raw honey. Stir, and let it sit for a few minutes. Sip slowly while you eat four edible flowers.

**At Sunset: Prepare another Ali's Breakfast Shake.**

Add two teaspoons of bee pollen to this one. Also, use an alternate protein powder if possible. It is always good to alternate protein powders, so you can digest them without difficulty.

Afterward, prepare two cups of hot saffron tea. Drink outside, and get plenty of deep breaths and the last of the sunshine on your body. Saffron tea has been proven to balance brain chemistry and significantly decrease cravings.

**Remember**: Please use no more than a pinch of saffron in each cup. If your food cravings persist, I advise drinking another Sleepy Time Tonic.

Before the next day's breaking of the fast, follow the morning instructions for Day 2. Then, prepare one last Bee Pollen Breakfast Blend. Enjoy the rest of your day!

**An Excellent "Breaking the Fast" Meal**

Enjoy a large, healthy, organic soup. It should contain vegetables and protein components. This soup should contain NO allergens such as gluten or dairy products.

Lentil soup, black bean soup, and cayenne pepper with squash are all acceptable.

**Breathing on a Mylar Blanket**

If you wish to extend your fast, lie on a Mylar blanket on the ground, with a blindfold over your eyes. A Mylar blanket will conduct free electrons from the earth's telluric field, and you will therefore be grounding without getting dirty.

Practice limbic breathing without moving for at least thirty minutes. Be still. Pay attention to your breath. You may want to blindfold yourself. Feel yourself in good health. Start to focus on the sensual feeling of wellness. You should be intensely relaxed and very focused this whole time. Do not fall asleep. Stay motivated, and complete thirty minutes of this exercise. When the thirty minutes are up, take the time to congratulate yourself!

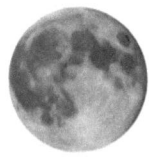

# Take The Pyramid Author's Challenge

If you are a young doctor or health coach aspiring to write a book, I offer you this challenge.

Write a manuscript, of at least sixty pages, reinterpreting my Holistic Health Pyramid from your perspective. Your topics may include, but are certainly not limited to, women's health, hormone health, sustainable home and health, animal health, health history, health futures, environmental awareness, autobiographical interpretations of health, health messages in story form, global health, community health, spiritual wholeness and health, addiction, longevity, or combinations thereof. My Holistic Health Pyramid, in its original and copyrighted form, must be displayed on the front page or back cover of your book with proper written attribution to me. Electronic books will be accepted.

The deadline for this project is May 25, 2015. All who submit manuscripts will be mentioned in my later books. I will select three winners. For each winner, I will write an introduction for your book. For the second-place writer, I will donate five hundred dollars to help you begin publishing or self-publishing your book. For the first-place writer, I will donate five hundred dollars to your publishing, as well as offer you a chance to accompany me as a guest speaker to one or more annual health fairs and festivals.

We all have a story in our pyramid. I would love to read yours. Help me share the magic of the Holistic Health Pyramid, while you seize the opportunity to enhance your career, writing talents, and personal education.

With all my best regards,

*Anthony James Canelo*

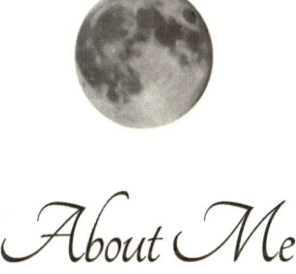

# About Me

I was raised in a health conscious family. My mother placed emphasis on conventional education *and* personal freedom. My father taught me how to ignore the world in order to follow my dreams. Through my teenage years I suffered from undiagnosed Epstein Barr syndrome, chronic fatigue, years of chronic primary insomnia, constant throat, ear, and skin infection, and ultimately a full blown case of shingles. At 18, my shingles transformed into an uncomfortable case of long-term post herpetic neuralgia; a nerve condition felt in the arms and throat. As a result of my condition, I could no longer articulate certain sounds. My hands and arms, sometimes paralyzed, always felt pain. I dropped out of school. Defeated in body and soul, I passed the time reading books in my room. While reading, living in my own world for over three years with old jazz and blues records, I licked my wounds and discovered I had nothing to lose.

My first landmark change was to stop abusing my mind with television. After that, I stopped abusing my body with medication. At 21, I began to fast, diet, yoga, and zealously research the health sciences. Observing myself get well was sobering and incredibly liberating. Naturally, I sought to improve other areas of my life. As time went by I gained many rich experiences in recovery and personal healing.

More than anything, I still desire to learn from the irreverent wisdom of my 21 year old self; a young man who found it so incredibly easy to release himself from his past and walk toward a brighter unknown. The day I'm gone, this is how I would like to be known. I am a graduate, health educator and recognized speaker of the Hippocrates Health Institute as well as a Certified Natural Health Professional (CNHP) by the Trinity

College of Natural Health. I teach workshops on health, sustainability and disaster preparedness. I have reversed my long term post-herpetic neuralgia, a known 'irreversible' nervous system condition. I have enjoyed my first unmedicated sleep in seven years. Today I proudly manage a holistic healing center, The Phoenix Institute of Holistic Health and Research, in Montclair, New Jersey. I am politically active and support the empowerment of all people.

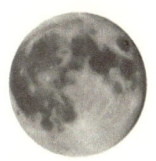

*Thank you so much for your inspiration, encouragement, and support.*

Emily Canelo, Peter Canelo, Nicholas Canelo, Cheryl Stoll-Thygerson Charles Walters, Russell Ditchfield Agboe, Dr. Brian Clement, Kazim Mirza, Paul Mantel, Bill Cameron, Matthew Mantel, Avery Mantel, Viktoras Kulvinskas, Ryan Monay, Danah Alexander, Myrlis Conde, Theodore Nathan, Kristen Boyer, Mike Jagger, Charles Walters, Douglas Drummond, Gail Barnett, Lucia Rose Horan, Andrew Goor, Matthew Chambers, Monique Lussier, Rupert Sheldrake, Ramtha, and JZ Knight.

The Five Rhythms Dance Community of New York City, WBAI 99.5 FM, New York City and their listenership, and the NDNS Family.

143